Your Guide to
Medical Hypnosis

LYNN PHELPS, M.D.

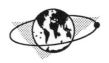

MEDICAL PHYSICS PUBLISHING
Madison, Wisconsin

Published by:

Medical Physics Publishing
732 N. Midvale Boulevard
Madison, WI   53705
(608) 262-4021

ISBN: 0-944838-28-6

Library of Congress Cataloging-in-Publication Data

Phelps, Lynn , 1926-
    Your guide to medical hypnosis / Lynn Phelps.
       p.   cm. -- (Focus on health)
    Includes bibliographical references and index.
    ISBN   0-944838-28-6 : $9.00
    1. Hypnotism -- Therapeutic use.
    2. Hypnotism -- Popular works.
  I. Title. II. Series: Focus on health (Madison, Wis.)
RC498.P49   1993
615.8 ' 512--dc20   93-9545
                                    CIP

Cover design by Mary Robertson

Foreword

The pendulum associated with the recognition of hypnosis has now swung towards acceptance. Few if any clinical applications have been given greater credibility towards these phenomena. Many questions as to how and why it is effective remain. The clinical results in this field are ahead of the laboratory. Noted pioneers in the field such as Mesmer, Braid, Esdaile, Charcot and Bernheim all gave credibility to this field. More contemporary researchers and clinicians such as Erickson, Hilgard, Spiegel and Orne have added credence to the field during this century. All of the pioneers and their disciples demonstrated the practical significance of using hypnotic phenomena and techniques in a patient population.

Often the term hypnosis conjures up much skepticism even from some medical and psychological colleagues. There are many "mythunderstandings" about the nature and use of hypnosis. The results of hypnosis are often perceived as being a result of either psychological or placebo factors. Research has shown that hypnosis goes beyond what experimenters might expect to obtain from these factors.

The ability to use hypnosis is a natural occurring phenomenon that each individual possesses. It is a misconception that one individual is possessed by another. The patient has the gift to utilize this power of concentration and discipline and thus is able to enter the altered state. Entering this altered state can facilitate changes in physiological and psychological responses. The gift of hypnosis is inherent in the individual. The doctor simply sets the stage for the patient to enter this altered state. The patients are helped to maximize their ability to utilize their talents.

A strategy is frequently supplied by the doctor in order to accomplish the above.

Many have feared that hypnosis permits the patient to be out of control. In reality, the patient obtains greater control and can participate in their own health care. Patients can then learn to decrease their dependence on medication, anesthesia and even doctor visits. They become more dependent on themselves and use the clinician to supply or develop effective strategies as well as make appropriate referrals when necessary.

Dr. Phelps' book **Your Guide to Medical Hypnosis** provides the reader with a practical introduction to this field. Through his own background and practices he provides excellent clinical examples that either he or other experienced clinicians have successfully used. A history of hypnosis along with the necessary steps to facilitate a patient's entering the altered state is provided. Dr. Phelps demonstrates the myriad of areas in medicine where hypnosis has been effective. Some of these areas include pain control, mastering of habits, alleviation of nausea and vomiting subsequent to chemotherapy or pregnancy, alleviation of phobias, etc. This guide will add to the literature that reduces the skepticism regarding this field as well as add invaluable support to the use of hypnosis in medicine.

Harold J. Wain, Ph.D.
Director, Consultation Liaison Psychiatry Clinic,
Walter Reed Army Medical Center,
Washington, D.C.

Professor, Department of Psychiatry,
Uniformed Services University of the Health Sciences,
School of Medicine,
Bethesda, Maryland

Preface

I once thought that hypnosis was used only to entertain an audience. I pictured someone with a pendulum or whirling lights putting some unwary soul under a spell to make him act like a fool. Seeing a fellow citizen bark like a dog, act like a chicken, or be unable to recognize someone in his family would certainly be amusing. But an exhibition like this would be at the expense of the person being hypnotized and essentially for the glorification of the hypnotist!

During my medical career in family practice, I learned that hypnosis can be used by doctors to help their patients. Habit disorders, problems with pain, insomnia, sexual dysfunction, and various phobias such as fear of flying can all be helped with medical hypnosis.

In medical hypnosis, there is no audience to be entertained. The doctor teaches the patient to use hypnosis for the patient's benefit without putting him or her under the doctor's control. In medical hypnosis, it is the patient who benefits.

Medical hypnosis made sense to me, so I began studying hypnotherapy in 1958 to learn to use hypnosis for my patients. In my busy family practice I began using medical hypnosis, not as a far-out type of therapy, but as a regular and routine means of helping patients. I attended many seminars and read numerous books and articles in the medical journals to help develop my skills. Over the years, I have been richly rewarded by being able to help many of my patients using the techniques I have learned.

This book will tell you about many of the medical uses of hypnosis. I will give examples of the use of hypnosis by some of the most successful clinical hypnotherapists in the world. I will discuss the four basic steps for successful therapy using medical hypnosis. I will describe the use of hypnosis in many medical, surgical, and psychological specialties. I will also describe how you can use hypnosis in your daily life. My hope is that you will find this book useful and that it will help you understand the many uses of medical hypnosis. Remember that hypnosis is an inexact science and most therapists using hypnosis in a clinical setting have developed their own theories and ideas on the subject. A perceptive reader of this and other books on the subject will note many differences in techniques, observations, and explanations as to what hypnosis is and what it can do. The ideas I present in this book naturally relate to my own study and experiences in the use of clinical hypnosis.

There is still much to be learned about the mind, especially about how the therapist can use various techniques, including medical hypnosis, for the benefit of the patient.

Lynn Phelps, M.D.

Acknowledgements

I wish to acknowledge Dr. John Cameron and Julie Bogle as well as Eileen Healy for their encouragement and helpful suggestions in the preparation of this book. Without their assistance it would not have been written.

Thanks also to my daughter, Ann Stone, whose pictures were taken by her husband, Tom Stone, and used in this book to demonstrate hypnosis in pregnancy. It may be of interest to readers that she used self-hypnosis during the labor and delivery of both of her children.

I also wish to acknowledge the artwork of my niece, Mary Robertson, who provided the drawings for the book's cover and chapter headings.

Gladys Meier and Barbara Sandrick edited and proofread the book.

I also appreciate the support of my wife, Sally.

Contents

CHAPTER 1

A Brief History of Hypnosis in Medicine

The first use of hypnosis as a medical treatment is lost in antiquity. Hypnotic techniques have been used since prehistoric times, but have been called by many different names. Early writers of Scripture were

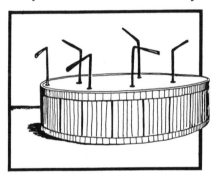

apparently aware of the powers of induced sleep, a form of hypnotic trance, as were people of other ancient civilizations. The Bible contains several references to the induction of sleep as a form of anesthesia.

Greek religion and mystical healing techniques made ample use of suggestions as part of therapy. An entire cult of temple healing developed as an adjunct to the worship of Asklepios, the god of healing and the son of Apollo. During *incubation* or *temple sleep* the patient slept or perhaps entered a trance so that the god Asklepios could appear to him in a dream and tell him that he would awake healed or give him instructions as to what he should do. Temple sleep seems to have allowed suggestions in a psychologically receptive state of mind. Medical hypnosis also gives suggestions to a psychologically receptive mind.

Similar practices, with strong religious overtones as part of the therapy, continued through the dark and middle ages. Even kings were credited with magical powers to treat loyal subjects. Whether the treatment involved medically useless potions or herbs really didn't matter if the subject had enough faith in the purveyors of the treatment. Certainly the medicine man of many societies used and continues to use faith as a healing mechanism. The hypnotic trance is a vital part of this form of therapy.

Mesmerism, named after Franz Anton Mesmer, was the first term used to describe the phenomenon we now call hypnosis. Mesmer was born in 1734 in Iznang, Germany. This was in the period between the Renaissance and the Enlightenment. He was well-educated, having studied Latin, music, philosophy, theology, mathematics, physics, and jurisprudence. Finally he studied medicine in Vienna. During his quest for information regarding types of influences on the mind, he came upon the ancient lore of planetary influences. Basing his argument on the known effects of sun and moon upon tides, seasons, and atmospheric conditions, he developed a theory. This theory stated that the heavenly spheres emit a fluid that penetrates everything and acts directly upon all the parts of a living organism. Mesmer believed that the nervous system was particularly sensitive to this fluid. After about 12 years of brooding on the idea that there was some sort of therapeutic power that could be passed from one person to another, he introduced the idea of *animal magnetism* . He believed that animal magnetism had therapeutic value and could be passed from one person to another. Although his studies and interpretations of the results of suggestion were later shown to be incorrect, they led to the modern science of hypnosis.

Mesmer left Vienna and went by a circuitous route to Paris, arriving there in 1778. He published a treatise titled *Mémoires sur la découverte de Magnetisme animal* in 1779. This publication created quite a sensation and a good deal of professional opposition. His work included the idea that a therapist could treat various ailments by simply passing a hand near the patient's head since the hand possessed the almost magical property of animal magnetism.

Mesmer's work later led to the use of therapeutic magnetized iron filings in a vat. Groups of patients, primarily women (see figure at the beginning of chapter one), would grasp the protruding iron rods and would enter a sort of trance, at times responding to the point of having convulsions or orgasms. In 1784 King Louis XVI of France was finally prevailed upon to appoint a commission to study Mesmer's claims. Members of the commission included Dr. Guillotin, designer of the guillotine, and Benjamin Franklin, the American scientist-diplomat, who was in France at the time. The commission studied Dr. Mesmer's writings and came to the conclusion that there was no scientific basis for the concept of animal magnetism. Mesmer was branded a quack and a charlatan. He retired into obscurity and, at the outbreak of the French Revolution, left France for England. It is interesting that even now in France, the word *magnetism* is used to describe hypnosis.

Although Dr. Mesmer dropped into obscurity, his ideas persisted. The transformation of mesmerism to modern hypnosis was gradual, and many physicians were involved. Two British doctors, John Elliotson and James Braid, became involved with mesmerism in the 1820s and treated many types of disorders with it. It is to Dr. Braid that we owe the terms *hypnosis* and *hypnotism*, which he used in place of mesmerism. He gave mesmerism a respectable physiological foundation, attributing the phenomenon to the effects of suggestion.

The famous French neurologist Jean Martin Charcot demonstrated that all manifestations of hysteria could be produced in hypnotized patients. Sigmund Freud was impressed with Charcot's findings and used hypnosis in his early years, only to abandon it as he developed his theories on psychoanalysis.

Following World War I and World War II, interest in hypnotherapy greatly increased when doctors discovered that it was useful in treating shell shock. The hypnotic trance was used both to eliminate symptoms directly and to treat soldiers who had repressed memories of traumatic battle situations. Under hypnosis, soldiers were able to recall various situations, relive them—sometimes with very strong emotional responses—and gradually improve.

In 1949 the Society of Clinical and Experimental Hypnosis was founded in the United States. Its members include physicians and scientists interested in further research in the phenomenon of hypnosis. The Society became international in 1959. A second society called the American Society of Clinical Hypnosis was founded in 1957. Its 3,000 members are primarily practicing psychiatrists, psychologists, dentists, and physicians of various specialties. In 1958, the American Medical Association and the American Dental Association made policy statements recognizing hypnosis as a legitimate form of treatment in medicine and dentistry. In 1960, the American Board of Medical Hypnosis was established to certify practitioners trained in the use of hypnotic suggestions.

Ernest and Josephine Hilgard (deceased) contributed significantly to the scientific research of hypnosis. Both received doctoral degrees at Yale, he in experimental psychology and she in child psychology. Their careers at Stanford University have been unique in that they studied many of the fundamental aspects of hypnosis using students as subjects. They are particularly well known for their studies regarding hypnosis and pain.

Dr. Milton H. Erickson is acknowledged as the prime promoter of modern clinical hypnosis. He was the founding president of the American Society of Clinical Hypnosis. He introduced the use of hypnotic techniques to many physicians, psychologists and dentists beginning in the late 1950s. My own interest in hypnosis began as a result of attending one of his seminars in 1958. Dr. Erickson died in 1980. His obituary stated that he had hypnotized 30,000 people during his career. A foundation for hypnosis research has been initiated in his honor. Dr. Erickson's contributions to the medical literature regarding the clinical uses of hypnosis are outstanding. The American Society of Clinical Hypnosis provides monthly seminars for training in hypnosis in the United States through its Education and Research foundation. It also conducts annual scientific meetings.

Although few medical schools offer extensive courses in the use of hypnotherapy, hypnosis research is being conducted at centers throughout the world. Every major city has practicing hypnotherapists, and interest in hypnosis continues to increase. Perhaps a time will come when hypnotic techniques will be a routine part of all medical and psychiatric therapies and all physicians will use hypnosis on a daily basis.

CHAPTER 2

Types of Therapists Who May Use Medical Hypnosis

Medical hypnosis is one of many techniques a doctor might use in caring for a patient. Any treatment, whether surgery, electroshock treatment, or the prescribing of medication, must be done by a well-trained professional. Hypnosis is no exception. The how, when, and why to use hypnosis must be a part of the training of the hypnotherapist.

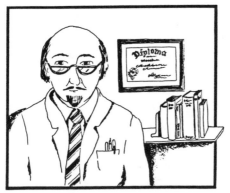

There are, however, few laws regulating the use of hypnosis. California and Florida are the only states with laws relating to the medical use of hypnosis. Unfortunately, some people call themselves medical hypnotists with little or no training other than in basic hypnotic techniques. They might advertise in the newspapers or in the yellow pages of the telephone book. There are many "institutes" that give certificates in hypnosis to people who have had only a small amount of training. These people may look very official but you should beware of the unscrupulous person passing himself or herself off as a hypnotist. You can always call local medical or psychological societies to check on a hypnotherapist's credentials. Also, there is nothing wrong in simply asking a person using hypnosis what his or her credentials are.

I checked on one such therapist at the request of a patient and found that she had finished high school and then took a basic course in hypnotic techniques. She set up shop and became quite successful; however, she had no basic medical or psychological training and her patients were at risk for developing psychological problems after hypnosis therapy.

Medical licensure in all states allows physicians to use procedures for which they have been trained. Psychologists and psychiatric social workers are also licensed or certified by the states in which they practice. Hospitals require physicians and surgeons to document their capability prior to practicing in the hospitals, but what doctors do in their offices comes under the states' licensing policies. This means that family physicians, pediatricians, internists, neurologists, and all members of the other specialties can use hypnotherapy for their patients providing they have a medical license and are trained to do so.

Psychiatrists are doctors with medical degrees who occasionally use hypnotherapy. They care for patients with mental disorders ranging from simple anxiety or depression to serious conditions such as schizophrenia.

Physicians in any specialty can obtain training in hypnosis through seminars or post-graduate courses. Few take the time to become trained as medical hypnotists, but nearly all specialties have doctors qualified to do hypnotherapy. The American Society of Clinical Hypnosis has a list of doctors who have taken courses through its educational branch.

Psychologists are not medical doctors but are trained in caring for persons with various types of mental disorders, including depression, anxiety, phobias, personality disorders, and family problems. Psychologists frequently use hypnotherapy for their patients. Psychologists have Ph.D. degrees and are therefore referred to as doctors.

Psychiatric social workers, specially trained nurses, members of the clergy, and other professionals may also use hypnotherapy within the limits of their training. Their techniques may vary considerably but you may find any of these professionals using medical hypnosis.

Some dentists are trained to use hypnosis for pain control, anxiety control, and control of secretions. Although they seldom advertise themselves as hypnotists, dentists with training in hypnotic techniques can be found by contacting your local dental society or the American Society of Clinical Hypnosis.

Hypnosis is a useful form of therapy for treating many medical and psychological conditions, but the hypnotherapist must use it within his or her own field. It is not an end in itself and can be misused just like any other form of therapy.

CHAPTER 3

Essentials of Hypnosis

Although there are various ways of describing mental activities, I find the simplest concept to be that of three basic categories: the conscious mind, the subconscious mind and the unconscious mind.

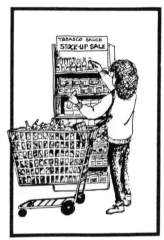

We are born with certain inherited abilities to function with the use of our *unconscious* minds. An example is the act of breathing, which occurs at the time of birth and does not require conscious effort or learned response.

Your *conscious* mind can make decisions. It can rationalize and weigh several alternatives and decide on the best one. The conscious mind is like the tip of an iceberg. It extends above the water but is only a very small part of the total mass of ice.

The *subconscious* mind is vast, like the part of the iceberg that is underwater. It is not easily accessible. Our past experiences are stored in the subconscious. Some investigators feel that everything we have ever learned is stored in the subconscious and is retrievable. Others feel that only the more important events in our lives are stored. Sometimes we can remember events or names and sometimes we can't. Sometimes we try to remember and only after changing the subject does the event or name reach our conscious minds. At times we recall events we feel we have long forgotten. We dream in the subconscious. Our feelings are primarily in the subconscious. Our daydreams originate in the subconscious. Our subconscious minds house our basic personalities and the essence of what is our true selves.

The subconscious cannot rationalize as can the conscious. It cannot reason and decide what is best. Since our subconscious minds cannot think in the conscious sense, they respond to ideas as though they are true, how ridiculous the ideas may seem. That's why no matter a dream can turn into a nightmare and have such strong effects. A deeply hypnotized person will swear that the sky is brown if such a suggestion is made and accepted. He or she will talk to a person who isn't present or, under the power of suggestion, will insist no one is in the room when it is actually filled with people.

The subconscious cannot rationalize but it can be influenced by suggestions from the conscious. Actually, it is being influenced all the time by what we see and hear; what we feel, taste and smell. A suggestible person is influenced, unknowingly, by advertisements and by remarks by friends. Personally, I am greatly influenced by casual comments made by friends and relatives. Since I am aware of it, I can make conscious decisions based on this knowledge, overriding my subconscious.

Another concept of importance is that of creativity. It is present in everyone. You may have a difficult problem to solve. You have tried to think of all the possible solutions, but have come up with a series of blanks. The solution may occur in your subconscious mind and may be blocked by prejudices of the past. Simply allowing your subconscious to work on the problem will frequently bring new ideas to your conscious mind.

Alternate States of Mind

In addition to these three basic categories of the mind, we can consider subdivisions of the subconscious as alternate states of the mind. Sleeping is one of the alternate states. Studies have shown that sleep is not merely the lack of consciousness, but is a complex state that varies considerably in depth and mental activity. Changes in the *EEG (electroencephalogram)*, (which measures the electrical pulses of the brain) distinguish types and varying depths of sleep. Night terrors, nightmares, somnambulism (sleepwalking), and sleep paralysis may occur during sleep. Dreams reveal our thoughts while sleeping. What lies between the complexities of conscious thought and the complexities of sleep?

Among the alternate states which occur naturally are two mental states which have strange sounding names. The *hypnogogic* state is that time just before falling asleep; the *hypnopompic* state occurs just before awakening.

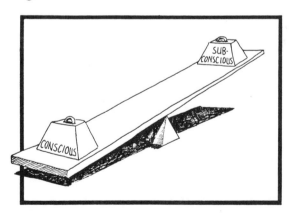

Alternate states of mind are *induced* by one means or another including yoga, transcendental meditation, progressive relaxation and hypnosis. While experiencing such mental states, a person is using both the conscious and subconscious minds at the same time, with one or the other having greater influence at any given time. The *depth of trance* is a measure of whether the conscious or subconscious part of the mind has more influence. As the influence of one goes up, the other goes down. One might think of it as a teeter totter. As the subconscious, representing one end of the teeter totter, goes up, the conscious, representing the other end, goes down. In deeper trance states the subconscious mind has greater control. Alternate states of mind are perfectly normal. Discussions of yoga, transcendental meditation and progressive relaxation are discussed in other books. I will limit my discussion to hypnosis.

Three Methods of Producing Hypnosis

Hypnosis is produced in one of three ways. First is *automatic hypnosis (autohypnosis)*. Autohypnosis occurs without a specific induction or formula. It occurs spontaneously by the act of concentrating on something such as a good book or movie. It also includes the automatic response to stimuli such as automatically looking toward a telephone which has rung. Our minds enter the automatic trance state when we drive and become unaware of our surroundings.

The second method of inducing hypnosis is by *heterohypnosis*, that is, by another person. A hypnotist need not be present—his or her voice may be recorded, or the person may be on the radio or television. The hypnotist may not even use words. If it is apparent to the subject that he or she should enter a trance state, this may be accomplished with no words spoken. I recall a seminar speaker who hypnotized several people by simply suggesting induction of a trance by his movements and touch.

The third method is *self-hypnosis,* or the intentional self-induction of hypnosis. Self-hypnosis will be discussed in more detail in Chapter 6.

The Value of the Subconscious Mind

We enter light trances every day of our lives. Sometimes when we go to a grocery store and reach for the various items on our lists, we think about the quality of the particular product as well as its cost and compare similar products. On other occasions, however, we simply slip into autohypnosis and our subconscious minds direct our hands to reach automatically for a specific product without really thinking about it. This automatic type of shopping is what advertisers aim for! In fact, our minds may be miles away thinking about the birthday dinner that we have to prepare or what we plan to do that evening. When we are done, our grocery baskets may be pretty full even though we did not give much real thought to how they got that way. When we automatically reach for items we are consciously thinking about something else. Our subconscious minds are in control and we are in an autohypnotic trance.

Actually, it is wonderful that we can let that vast subconscious part of the mind function on its own since most of what we do in our everyday lives is automatic. If we had to think how to get up from a seated position, how to put one foot in front of the other to walk, how to get into a car, how to drive, and how to maneuver inside a store, we wouldn't get anything else done. Once we have learned to do an activity, we can store the knowledge away in our subconscious minds and just perform it automatically the next time. That is what learning is all about.

On the other hand, the conscious part of our mind is limited. What we are thinking and deciding to do at any particular moment is only a tiny part of what is going on in our minds. Another example of conscious versus subconscious activity is the route I take to work every day. If I follow my usual route, my subconscious mind knows the way and I drive to work without thinking much about it. If, on the other hand, I decide to take an alternate route due to construction or simply for a change of scenery, I must consciously think as I drive so that I eventually get to the proper place.

The Trance State

Hypnosis makes use of an *alternate state of consciousness*. One such alternate state of mind is the *trance state*. A trance state isn't something exotic or magical, but simply something that happens all the time to everyone. In a trance state any thought, action or other response to an idea comes from the subconscious rather than from the conscious mind. This opens up all sorts of possibilities.

To define a trance in more medical terms, it is the alternate state of mind in which the subconscious responds directly to stimuli, whether heard, seen or felt. The induction of a trance state is simply the use of our subconscious minds for a specific purpose.

There are various depths of a trance, from simply reaching subconsciously for a favorite product to a deep somnambulistic trance state in which a person acts as though he or she is asleep. A somnambulistic trance state is deeper and longer lasting than a light trance. It has a more specific beginning and end.

While a light trance is simply a subconscious response to any stimulus, a more prolonged trance, or trance state, continues for a longer period of time. The terms trance and trance state do not have precise definitions and are used differently by different writers. I like to think of the term trance as including any subconscious response to a stimulus. A light trance would include the spontaneous responses described previously. Deeper trances last for longer periods; I term these trance states. Trance states may last as long as a movie or a television show, a sporting event, the reading of a book, or the act of daydreaming.

We often enter a trance state when we go to a movie. As we enter the theater we anticipate seeing something enjoyable, scary, funny, or tragic depending on what we know about the film. As we settle down (probably with popcorn, which we tend to buy automatically), we become entranced with the action on the screen. We gradually enter a deep spontaneous trance state of autohypnosis as we begin to get involved with what we see on the screen. Gradually the person next to us fades away, and the people in front of us also fade away unless they are talking or are wearing big hats. We may laugh, cry, move with the action, shiver with horror, or break out in a sweat. In effect we become a part of the action. The more we become involved with the action, the deeper our trance state. At the end of the movie, it sometimes takes us several minutes to come out of the trance state.

Children are very good at entering trances and participate in rather prolonged automatic trance states on frequent occasions. Perhaps you can remember watching a child playing house with dolls and teddy bears, completely unaware of his or her actual surroundings. I recall watching my grandson having a birthday party for one of his teddy bears. All of the stuffed animals that were at the party had names and my grandson talked to them as though they were alive. Presumably they talked back to him, as he seemed to be listening to them. To bring him out of the trance state I had to speak rather loudly to him. This activity is perfectly natural and normal for all of us, although children seem to be better at it.

Children are particularly susceptible to the trance state because they are very imaginative and have none of the hang-ups that we adults have about such things. With proper instruction, however, almost any of us can enter a trance state if there is a reason to do so. The reason may be anything from ridding oneself of a bad habit to controlling a chronic pain problem. This sounds a bit like "the power of positive thinking" and in a sense it is, but the approach is at both the conscious and subconscious levels of the mind. Since feelings, biases, fears, and memories reside in the subconscious, attacking them at that level through hypnosis makes sense. This is truly the basis for medical hypnosis. We can influence the conscious mind with logical ideas whereas we can influence the subconscious mind with ideas which may be quite illogical. Suggestions given while in the hypnotic trance state are accepted by the subconscious mind as being true no matter how ridiculous they may seem to the conscious mind. This is the framework within which the hypnotist is able to influence his patient.

The trance state is not a clearly defined state of mind with the subject either in a trance state or not in a trance state. It is actually a fluid, dynamic condition in which the trance level can vary from a very light to a very deep trance. I have previously discussed the light automatic trances. A subject passes through the light trance on the way to the deeper trance states. The deepest trance state is called the *somnambulistic* trance. This level is similar to sleepwalking. In a deep trance, one can walk, talk, see and act pretty much as in the waking state. Fortunately, deep trances are not necessary for hypnotic therapy. Hypnosis can be of great value even when only a light trance is produced; this means nearly everyone can benefit from hypnosis as a form of therapy.

Although most people can't enter deep trances, for some purposes the ability to do so is actually counterproductive to the use of hypnosis for therapy. A person who is very susceptible to hypnotic suggestion is also very susceptible to casual suggestions when not in the trance state. If a very susceptible person wishes to be a nonsmoker, the effects of the deep trance will be more helpful in the short run, but the chances of the subject taking a cigarette offered at a later time by a friend may be increased due to his or her greater susceptibility to suggestion. A less susceptible person might very well succeed in the long run while the more susceptible person might fail.

Susceptibility to Trance

No one really knows why some people are more susceptible to the hypnotic trance than others. We do, however, vary in our ability to enter the trance state. About five percent of us have trouble entering even light states, while another five percent of us can enter deep trances with no difficulty. I am not aware of any studies explaining these differences. Perhaps our susceptibility is something we are born with or perhaps it is a result of what we learn as infants. It is probably a combination of both. Perhaps we are better subjects if our mothers were good hypnotists. Some mothers spend a lot of time cuddling their babies, cooing to them, talking to them, rocking them, and in effect giving them hypnotic suggestions. Such repetitive sounds, soothing sounds, relaxing sounds, and monotonous repetitions are all useful in helping people go into deeper trances. Unfortunately, other mothers don't relate to their infants in this manner. Some mothers prop the bottle so the baby doesn't have human contact while being fed. Some feed the baby the bottle, but instead of interacting with the baby, watch TV or read a book or magazine. Perhaps the baby that is cuddled and talked to and has a strong interaction with the mother turns out to be a better hypnotic subject. Can we learn to be better hypnotic subjects with practice? Hypnotic ability follows a bell shaped curve.

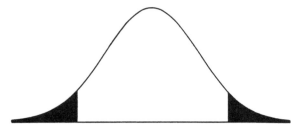

Ninety percent of people fall within the hypnotizable range. More people are at the middle of the curve; the numbers decrease towards the ends of the curve. Dr. Herbert Speigel from New York devised a system of classifying people on a numerical scale from one to five called the *Hypnosis Induction Profile*. People classed as one are those who find entering a hypnotic trance very difficult while those classed as five are those who seem to be in a trance most of the time because they are so susceptible! There is really no way to tell exactly where you would be classified on this scale without being tested. There are other types of hypnosis scales. The one most widely used for research in hypnosis is the *Stanford Profile Scale of Hypnotic Susceptibility*. A trained hypnotist can usually get a pretty good idea of susceptibility in about five or ten minutes.

Non-Medical Uses of Trance

Many uses of trance states have been found to be of value over the centuries. Yoga is one example. Entering a yoga trance requires concentration and involves spiritual and physical endurance. Another example of the trance state is transcendental meditation. Although the means of entering the trances and their purposes may be different, the ability of the mind to enter the trance state is the basis for success in both cases.

The hypnotic trance state is used for various purposes. As an example, the stage hypnotist uses the hypnotic trance state for entertainment. I remember my first experience with a stage hypnotist. I was in the army during World War II and one of the U.S.O. shows advertised a hypnotist as one of the acts. We all went to the performance eager to see what he would do to the poor "sucker" that he coaxed into being his subject. I had no idea what to expect, although I had heard that hypnotism was something some people could do to other people to cause them to make fools of themselves. The hypnotist's first act was to ask those interested in being subjects to come to the stage. Being young and curious, I was one of those who went. I quote from a letter I sent home at the time:

> About 10 chairs were placed in a semicircle. He took us to the center as individuals, and made us fall over backwards. I fell but fortunately he caught me! Then he made us clasp our hands

and asked us to make them so tight that we couldn't unclasp them. Some fun. Then we held our right arms out straight and couldn't bend them. Lastly, he tried to put us all asleep at once, but due to the interruption of the audience laughing when the WAAC fell over on me, I didn't go under. I nearly did a couple of times but not quite. About three actually were under his power, and he made them laugh, make funny faces, dance, change their shoes, and such. It was very funny, but I'm glad I didn't go out! It was all very interesting.

I remember that I was affected by his suggestions, but I was not susceptible enough to be one of the subjects for his show. Looking back on it, however, I can see that the technique he used to increase his credibility was to take subjects from the audience and to select those persons most susceptible to his suggestion. He put the three who were able to go into the deep trance states through their paces, suggesting that they do all sorts of interesting things to entertain the rest of us. Since we knew the people he used as his subjects, it was obviously not a hoax. I wondered at the time why they were able to act as his subjects and I was not. I didn't know anything about hypnotic susceptibility then. That experience, however, helped me become interested in the medical uses of hypnosis years later.

CHAPTER 4

The Four Basic Steps of Hypnotherapy

For the therapeutic hypnotic trance state, there must be four steps.

The First Step: Hypnotic Induction

The beginning of a hypnotic trance state is the attention-getter or *induction*. A subject must concentrate on something to begin to enter the trance state. While there are various induction techniques, I prefer the *eye roll induction*. This was introduced by Dr. Her-

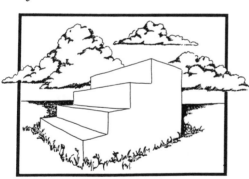

bert Speigel, a professor at Columbia University, both as an induction and as a quick way of determining a person's hypnotic susceptibility. It consists of having the subject roll the eyes upward as far as possible and then slowly close the eyelids over the upturned eyes. Dr. Speigel noted that as people entered a trance, their eyes tend to roll upward no matter what induction technique is used. He tested this phenomenon and noted that the more easily a person could roll the eyes up and the more often they stayed up while the eyelids were being closed, the more susceptible that person was to the hypnotic trance. Later, the eye roll was found to be only about 75% accurate as an indicator of hypnotizability.

Performing the eye roll, however, seems to work well as an induction technique no matter how susceptible a person is. It fulfills several needs of a successful induction. It reduces outside interference since the eyes are closed early. It fosters concentration on a specific act, that of rolling up the eyes. It also leads nicely to the second step, or deepening of the trance state.

There are other commonly used inductions. The subject can stare at a light source or a moving pendulum, into the eyes of the hypnotist or at a spot on the wall. The hypnotist then gives suggestions of relaxation and the eyelids becoming so heavy that they must close. In another approach, the subject is asked to think about one or both hands becoming very light and gradually rising from the lap. As the hands are rising, it is suggested that the eyelids are becoming heavy and will close.

Although there are many more induction techniques, the only other one I will describe is called the *Chiasson Technique*. Dr. Simon Chiasson, an Ohio obstetrician, noted that if a person extends the arm and stares at one of the knuckles, a suggestion that the fingers will gradually spread apart will cause them to do so. Suggestions are then made that the hand will automatically move toward the face and that the eyes will gradually close.

The specific induction technique that is used is of little consequence as long as it serves to begin the trance state. The process of induction can be accelerated by instructing the patient about the use of a *cue word* or *action*. A cue is suggested as part of the therapeutic aspect of the hypnotic trance and is useful for later inductions. An example of a cue word would be the word "relax." The therapist's pressing lightly on the patient's shoulder would be an example of a cue action. A cue for the induction of self-hypnosis might be the pressure of a thumb against an index finger.

The Second Step: Deepening the Trance

The second step in the therapeutic trance is called *deepening the trance.* A trance state might be light, moderate or deep. There are no distinct separations between these designations, but the patient's subconscious will accept ideas more readily while in the deeper stages of the trance. Suggestions used for deepening the trance depend on the personality of the subject. Each of us is particularly susceptible to certain types of suggestions or ideas which will help deepen the trance. Most people respond to simple suggestions of relaxation. Some people respond best to ideas related to visual imagery. A visual person responds primarily to ideas of seeing something in his or her imagination. An example would be the suggestion of watching a television program or a movie. You often hear this type of person referring to a comment by saying "I see what you mean." Other people respond better to suggestions regarding the sense of hearing. The hearing person responds best to ideas of hearing sound such as an orchestra or popular singing group. These people will often respond by saying "I hear what you are saying." Still others seem to respond best to the sense of feeling. The feeling person is the one who responds best to a bodily sensation such as feeling himself going down an elevator or escalator and may respond to a statement "I feel that you are on the right track." Some people respond well to suggestions of age regression and can readily revert in time to some previous age or activity and *relive* an experience much as it actually happened.

The length of time needed for deepening the trance depends on the subject's natural ability. Deepening may take only a few seconds or many minutes. The more a person practices, the easier and faster it will be to achieve a deeper trance, although the ultimate depth of the trance an individual achieves depends on his or her natural ability.

During my first appointment with you I would use a *test trance* to determine how you respond to various types of deepening suggestions. I do this by telling you that I will be giving several types of suggestions and that you will be able to tell me afterward which of the suggestions worked the best. I then use a simple induction such as the eye roll, followed by suggestions of relaxation. These suggestions might include having you visualize a rag doll with no bones or muscles lying on the floor. The mental image of a kitten lying in the sun completely relaxed and at ease might help you achieve a similar feeling of relaxation. At times the mental image of specific words helps. I say "As you hear me say certain words, your mind will form images of what those words mean to you." Then I use words such as tranquil, serene, peace, quiet, or more simply, relax. Relaxation itself is not a passive act, but something which a person must expend some energy to accomplish. You must consciously allow your muscles to be more passive. You can do this by feeling various bundles of muscle fibers giving way and then continuing to be devoid of tension.

Once you are relaxed, I give feeling, seeing, and hearing suggestions as I talk you down a path into a sunken flower garden. I give the a sense of motion, or feeling, by suggestions of walking down the path. Seeing the various flowers, trees, fountains and gravel path are visual images. Hearing the birds, wind in the trees, distant sounds of traffic or perhaps an airplane are examples of hearing sensations. There are countless suggestions I can use for the purpose of deepening the trance. Walking in the sand at the seashore, enjoying a sporting event, and seeing and hearing a concert are examples.

Next I use age regression suggestions. These take you mentally back in time a few hours, days, weeks, months or even years to an important or pleasant event in your life. I suggest that you relive the event in its fullness including the sights, sounds, smells, and tastes. I particularly suggest that you repeat the feelings associated with the original event. By this time, you may be in a moderate to deep trance state. The depth of the trance does not depend as much on the specific suggestions given as on your susceptibility to them.

I then suggest that you will be able to remember all that went on during the trance state and that you will arouse from the trance, continuing to be relaxed and at ease. I say that you can come out of the trance by the simple act of opening your eyes. I then ask which of the suggestions were the most realistic. I ask that you rate my suggestions on a scale of one to four, one being the least helpful and four being the most helpful. This gives me an idea as to which deepening suggestions will be the most helpful during therapy and also tells me how suggestible you are.

The Third Step: Therapeutic Suggestions

In the third step of hypnotherapy actual therapeutic suggestions are given. If you wish to become a nonsmoker, for example, I would give you positive suggestions toward that goal. If you had chronic pain I would give you suggestions that would lead to greater physical comfort. The person having trouble flying in an airplane would receive suggestions about the enjoyment of air travel. After these suggestions are made, the subconscious mind is urged to allow the suggestions to continue to be effective even after the formal trance state has ended.

Since the effect of the suggestions will last for a certain period following the trance and then gradually be lost, the suggestions I gave you must be reinforced. I prefer to make an audio-tape of the actual therapeutic hypnotic session and give it to you to take home. I suggest that you repeat the hypnotic trance with its therapeutic suggestions at least three times a day for a period of several weeks. I would also teach you self-hypnosis so that you can alternate self-hypnosis with the tape and eventually give up the tape and use self-hypnosis alone. In this way, you will have learned a new skill which can be used for many different purposes. In subsequent chapters, I will give more examples of therapeutic suggestions.

What makes hypnotherapy worthwhile is that part of the subconscious will continue to respond to the suggestions after the trance state is over. This phenomenon is referred to as *post hypnotic suggestion*. This effect may last only a few minutes, but more frequently lasts several days. This is the main value of hypnosis as a form of psychotherapy.

The Fourth Step: Arousal From the Trance

The final step in the therapeutic hypnotic trance is arousing from the trance state to consciousness. I suggest to you that at a certain cue the trance state will end. This can be accomplished in several ways. I may suggest that on the count of three the trance will be over, or I may simply suggest that the patient's eyes will open, ending the trance state. It may take several seconds or even minutes to end a deep trance. The suggestions given during the trance will continue to be effective. As an example, if I suggest that you will continue to be very relaxed and at ease after the trance is finished, you will tend to feel that way.

These, then, are the four steps of a therapeutic hypnotic treatment: induction, deepening, therapeutic suggestions, and arousal.

CHAPTER 5

Types of Therapeutic Suggestions

Let's say that you have broken your arm. The hypnotherapist can help you enter a trance state (induction) and then use various suggestions to deepen your trance (deepening techniques). You are in a receptive state, but the broken arm needs care and still hurts. At this point, one or more of the following types of therapeutic suggestions may be given to you: ideosensory, ideomotor, ideonominal, age regression,

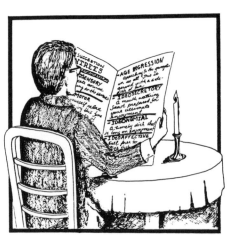

ideosecretory, ideoaffective or dissociation. I will explain each of these below. The therapist will decide which type of suggestions might be the most effective for you.

An *ideosensory suggestion* influences your subconscious mind to create a sensation. This sensation is then believed by your conscious mind to be true. Suggestions may relate to any of your five senses—sight, smell, touch, taste, or hearing. A suggestion of visual imagery would perhaps relate to your seeing a movie within your mind. Much like a dream, you would experience the sensation of seeing the movie rather than being in your doctor's office. Taste and smell suggestions might have you enjoying some popcorn at the show. A suggestion related to hearing might allow you to tune out the sounds of the doctor's office so that you could hear the sounds of the movie instead. In the meantime, the doctor can go ahead and treat your broken arm. He may inject numbing medicine into the fracture site if the trance state isn't deep enough for hypnotic anesthesia. If you are in a deep trance the doctor may be able to set the fracture and apply a cast with no other anesthesia.

While the subconscious mind can create the sensation of touch or feeling, it can also create a sensation of numbness. The absence of the sensation of touch is anesthesia. Major surgery has been performed using the hypnotic suggestion of "no pain" as the only anesthesia.

An *ideomotor suggestion* can cause a muscular action. Muscles move all the parts of our bodies. Hypnotic suggestion can cause your muscles to move even if you consciously wish them not to. An example of this is arm levitation. Arm levitation is simply the act of your arm slowly rising in the air in response to the suggestion that it will rise. The subconscious mind causes the arm to move even if your conscious mind is trying to prevent it. Another example is the suggestion that one of your fingers will move automatically without conscious effort. After a brief time, your finger will actually move. A variation of this phenomenon can be used in obtaining answers from your subconscious mind to questions related to your problem. A specific finger movement can indicate "yes" and another finger movement "no." Still another finger can be instructed to move if the answer is "I prefer not to answer" or "I don't know the answer."

The opposite of motion is lack of motion. Muscles are normally in the state of partial stimulation so that you can sit upright, stand or walk with no conscious effort. Even when you are asleep at night, you move many times. Ideomotor suggestions can cause the subconscious mind to completely relax certain muscles or even your whole body. Your broken arm is more easily treated with less pain when you are relaxed. Total relaxation leads to natural sleep if you have insomnia. Relaxation also helps if you are planning to take an examination or perform before an audience.

An *ideonominal suggestion* influences your perception of time. It can distort your sense of the passage of time, or cause the reliving of events from the past. An example of the first is that time flies when you are having fun. On the other hand, time really drags when you are in the dentist's chair undergoing a root canal. Ideonominal suggestions can create the perception that fun times seem long and enjoyable while unpleasant times seem short and endurable. This phenomenon is useful when a patient must endure a period of discomfort such as a bandage change.

Age regression is a type of idionominal suggestion. It is the term used for reverting subconsciously to an earlier time. When you regress to the second grade, you respond to questions as though you were actually seven years old. You write as you did at that age, and you remember what was happening in the schoolroom at that time. If you spoke a different language as a child, age regression may cause you to revert to your native tongue. In the treatment of your broken arm, diverting your attention to a fun time in your life through age regression could relieve you of worry about your arm.

Questions have been raised regarding the truth of memories obtained through age regression. On occasion, new information obtained by this method is verified by other means. On other occasions, however, information which seems to be true to the subject has proven to be false. In court cases, information obtained through the use of age regression must be verified by other sources.

The reaction to an *ideosecretory suggestion* is easy to understand when you think of a hamburger or steak cooking over a grill. Almost immediately, your mouth waters in anticipation of biting into such a feast. There are many organs and glands in the body that secrete fluids. The tear glands secrete tears that bathe the eye in a nutrient solution. Excess tears occur during crying or at times of extreme joy. Saliva is produced to begin the digestive process when you enjoy a meal. Nasal secretions are always present to moisten the nasal cavities, but with a common cold they may be excessive. The kidneys excrete water and chemicals that are not needed by the body. The pancreas secretes enzymes to aid in digestion, while the liver secretes many chemicals necessary for bodily function. The pituitary, thyroid, adrenals, ovaries, testicles, and other organs and glands also secrete various types of hormones necessary for the orderly function of your body. The ideosecretory response in hypnosis isn't used as much as other types of suggestion. If a dentist needs a patient to have a dry mouth, however, the suggestion of lack of saliva, using the ideosecretory response, can be used for this purpose.

An *ideoaffective suggestion* changes your *affect*, or attitude about a situation. Affect is defined as one's feelings, emotions, or desires. Although we like to think we have conscious control over our feelings, the real center of our emotions resides in our subconscious minds. We refer to "getting up on the wrong side of the bed" when we are in a bad mood. There are some days when we really wish we could have stayed in bed. Some days we feel "on top of the world" and only wish we had more time to enjoy the feeling. What determines how we feel about what's going on?

Many things do, of course. I remember being inspired by a woman with advanced cancer. One would expect her to be very depressed. Actually she continued writing poetry and was productive and upbeat in spite of her tragedy. I have also seen people who should be sitting on top of the world but are "down in the dumps." A recent event, such as breaking an arm, may be an important factor in how we are feeling. No one wants to be hurting and no one wants to be in a cast for four to five weeks. On the other hand, perhaps being in a cast will get you out of doing certain chores around the house that you don't like. Perhaps being in a cast will make a schoolboy a hero at school or even allow him to miss his dreaded rope climbing in gym. Most of the time we really don't know why we feel the way we do. The causes of elation and depression are usually deeply buried in the subconscious mind and they may be very hard to uncover.

In therapy, ideoaffective suggestions can be used to point out the advantages of a difficult situation. During the trance state, the suggestion can be made that one should feel good about one's accomplishments and advantages in spite of a particularly difficult situation. Such suggestions may make the acceptance of the situation much more bearable.

Dissociation refers to the sensation of being outside the body. Such a suggestion may give you the feeling that your mind is removed from your body. It may be in another part of the room or somewhere else entirely. If you believe that your mind is outside your body, you can't feel the pain your body is experiencing. This technique is particularly useful during childbirth.

Three Basic Laws of Psychology

The hypnotherapist must consider some basic psychological laws when deciding what types of suggestions to use in a particular situation. The *Law of Concentrated Attention* states that when your attention is concentrated on an idea, the idea tends to be realized. This means that when you think strongly about something, that something tends to happen. For example, if you are a smoker and think about having a cigarette, the more you think about it, the greater your chances of having one, even if you are in the process of giving up smoking. If you are overweight and you think about eating some candy, the Law of Concentrated Attention states that you will eventually have some, even if it means going out in the middle of the night to find a store.

The *Law of Reversed Effect* states that when willpower, which is in the conscious mind, and the imagination, which is in the subconscious mind, come into conflict, the imagination always wins. This is because the subconscious is more powerful than the conscious. According to the Law of Reversed Effect, even if you consciously say that you will NOT have that cigarette, your subconscious or imagination says, "Oh yes you will!" You will most likely find a way to have that cigarette.

The *Law of Dominant Effect* states that attaching an emotion to an idea makes the realization of that idea more likely. The stronger the emotion, the greater the likelihood of realization. As an example if you are studying for an exam, and your roommate suggests you go to the latest movie, your will power says, "No, I must study," but your subconscious says, "Hey, you studied last time and flunked anyway, so what the hell, let's go to the movie." Anyway, you have probably had a deep desire to see that particular movie because the advanced promotion fits in with some of your deepest feelings.

A Case Study Using Hypnotherapy

Examples of some of the principles of hypnotherapy as discussed above can be found in this paraphrase of a case study published by Drs. Erickson, Hershman, and Sector:

Mr. and Mrs. J., a young, very religious couple, came to the office most hesitantly, stating that their problem was that each of them wet the bed regularly. Briefly, their story was as follows: When they got married, each kept their bed wetting a secret from the other. The morning after their wedding night, they were both very polite and appreciative that the other didn't complain about the wet bed. For nine months, things went along in that manner. Then one of them said to the other that it would be nice if they had a baby on whom to blame the wet bed. That led to their discovery that they were both bedwetters. They continued to wet the bed every night for another three months before they made up their minds to seek therapy.

After Doctor Erickson met Mr. and Mrs. J. and learned their story he discovered that they had no money at all. An offer was made to treat them on an experimental basis. If he succeeded, his reward would be the satisfaction of curing them. If, however, they were not cured they were to be charged standard psychiatric fees.

While Mr. and Mrs. J. were in a very light hypnotic trance, they were asked to promise that they would obey all the instructions given to them, no matter how absurd, ridiculous, or outrageous they might seem. Their deep religious beliefs made it a certainty that they would obey a solemn promise. The instructions they were given were as follows: Every night they were to go to the toilet at six o'clock. They were to drink a glass of water before going to bed. They were to go to bed with the door to the bathroom locked. They would get into bed, kneel hand in hand facing their pillows on the bed, and proceed to urinate and get the necessary bed wetting over with. After that they could lie down with the certainty that the bed wetting had already been accomplished and be able to sleep the rest of the night without worrying about what time of the night they had wet the bed. They promised to do this for two weeks and were instructed that at the end of this time they could take a night's vacation; that is, they could go to bed without first wetting the bed. They were told that the morning after their vacation, if they saw a wet bed, they would know what to do next. They followed the instructions, and when the time came for their vacation, a Sunday night, they felt so happy to lie down in a dry bed that they slept all through the night without wetting the bed. After all, they had had two weeks of practice sleeping through the night without wetting the bed! When on Monday morning they threw back the covers and saw a dry bed, it left them rather confused. They had been instructed not to discuss matters with each other. As they described it later, since they didn't know what to do Monday night, they just turned off the light and sneaked into bed. They awoke on Tuesday with bed dry again. On Tuesday night, they sneaked into bed once more.

At the end of three weeks with a dry bed, they returned to the office. They had been told that they would return with an amazing story. When they arrived, they were still confused and uncertain about what had been happening to them. They had a dry bed for three whole weeks and, they said, they did not know what to do next. Seemingly casual matters were discussed with them for a while and then the statement was made, "Next month is May," and they were literally shoved out of the office. In May they returned to report that all was going well. A year later they came in proudly to introduce their baby, stating that now they could have a wet spot on their bed any time they wanted to, but it would be a cute little wet spot.

The indirect approach—not letting Mr. and Mrs. J. know his strategy, making them work for their own good, and forcing them into a situation in which they had a bed that they did not wet during their sleep—built up in them the realization that they could have a dry bed. Of course, during therapy they wet the bed before they went to sleep, but that was another matter entirely. That was a controlled act; they controlled it. They also controlled keeping the bed from being wet additional times during the night. Thus they learned to have a dry bed.*

In summary, the hypnotherapist can use several types of suggestions in helping a patient with a problem. The cigarette addict can be helped to feel upbeat, proud and happy as a nonsmoker and to enjoy the many benefits that not smoking brings. The person in chronic pain can be made more comfortable by suggestions of numbness, dissociation, relaxation and age regression. The person who fears flying can be given suggestions that let him or her feel the freedom that flying through the air allows and the exhilaration of being free of the confines of earth.

---

*Milton H. Erickson, M.D., Seymour Hershman, M.D. Irving I. Secter, D.D.S., *The Practical Application of Medical and Dental Hypnosis*, New York, adapted with permission from Bruner/Mazel

I use the various types of suggestions discussed in this chapter in various combinations for the greatest effect. My methods depend on my training and experience, naturally, and no two practitioners will treat you in exactly the same way. If one attempt at hypnotic therapy does not yield the desired effect, I usually suggest that you see another therapist. I have successfully treated patients who have failed with another hypnotist, and some of my patients have succeeded with another clinician after failing to be helped by me.

CHAPTER 6

Self-Hypnosis

I referred earlier to *self-hypnosis* and will now discuss it in more detail. How can you hypnotize yourself? The notion that the hypnotist actually hypnotizes you must be dropped. The hypnotist does not. He or she simply teaches you how to hypnotize yourself. This is an entirely different concept than forcing you to do something. You, the patient, must be willing to be hypnotized. You must want to explore your own subconscious mind. You come to me or another medical hypnotist to learn how to do it. You can also learn

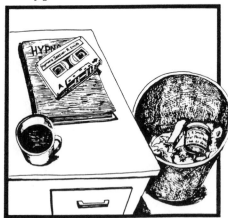

from a book, a cassette tape, or from a friend who has learned the techniques. There is nothing magical in how it's done.

Self-hypnosis is the conscious manipulation of the subconscious part of the mind. Since the subconscious cannot "think," it responds to ideas as though they are true, no matter how ridiculous they may be. In self-hypnosis, your conscious mind and your subconscious mind are in communication. Since your subconscious mind is very *literal*, you must be careful what your conscious mind suggests. If you suggest that something is sickening, you may vomit. If you have a fear of elevators and suggest to yourself that you are riding in one, you may break out in a cold sweat. On the other hand, if you suggest that you have no concerns, you will relax. If you suggest that you go back in time and relive a pleasant experience, you can ignore a painful situation such as a dental drill. If you fear that you will do badly on an examination and block on the answers, you can use self-hypnosis to relax and let your knowledge flow freely.

During self-hypnosis, your conscious mind directs certain thoughts and your subconscious mind responds. This process resembles a dialogue between two people but it actually occurs within your own mind. There is no need for you to say the suggestions out loud. You can simply say them to yourself and wait for a response before proceeding.

The trance state is usually not as deep in self-hypnosis as in heterohypnosis since in self-hypnosis the hypnotist and the subject are the same person. The conscious mind usually cannot relinquish its control to the extent that it occurs in the heterohypnotic trance. Self-hypnosis amounts to the conscious mind giving ideas to the subconscious and the subconscious responding. The response may be perceived sensations or movement of the parts of the body. You might think of it as a conversation between two parts of the brain.

During self-hypnosis your conscious mind can direct your subconscious to change. The change is presumably for the better! An example would be a change in your feelings. When you get up "on the wrong side of the bed," you would probably rather be in a good mood. You can hypnotize yourself and suggest to your subconscious mind that you prefer to be in a good mood. You can stress the good things in life and ignore the bad. It's as though you went back to bed and "got up on the right side."

I have used this technique in the past to good

advantage. I remember using it before attending a social function on one occasion. I liked the company of the hosts, but didn't particularly like some of their friends. I really didn't want to go. My wife and I had accepted the invitation, however, and I decided to try to alter my feelings by the use of self-hypnosis. After a brief induction, I suggested to my subconscious that I would enjoy myself and have a good time in spite of who might be there. Actually, I had a ball. I played the piano for a sing-along and sang loudest of all. I had a wonderful time. On the way home I told my wife what an enjoyable evening it had been. Her comment was, "It was obvious you were having a good time. You certainly made an ass of yourself doing so!" Fortunately for me she was smiling when she made her comment.

I'll explain briefly how I personally go about using self-hypnosis. I begin self-hypnosis by using a cue to enter a trance. The cue is to press my right thumb and index finger together. It is a cue that I learned many years ago and has always served me well. As I enter the trance state, my thumb and finger relax. I then deepen my trance by age regressing to a sailing trip in the Virgin Islands. I see the sailboat, sense the wind, and feel the boat moving up and down through the waves. Depending on my mood at the time, I might use a different deepening suggestion such as entering a warm, comfortable room with a fire in the fireplace. Soon I am in a comfortable trance state and am ready for other suggestions. I frequently suggest that when I am in a deep enough trance for a beneficial effect, one of my fingers will move automatically. Then I wait for my finger to move. Sometimes it happens rapidly and sometimes it takes a while. If I get no response, I start over. The reasons for my self-hypnosis may vary from getting to sleep after a hectic day at work to relaxing prior to a meeting that I know will be stressful. I may use it merely to relax and remove myself for a time from the activities of the day. It is easier, cheaper, and healthier than a double martini, with or without the olive. At times it works rapidly and well. On rare occasions it doesn't seem to work at all. Sometimes the suggestions are accepted by my subconscious and at other times they are rejected. My suggestions work more often than not although I don't consider myself to be a particularly susceptible subject.

I have mentioned some of the reasons I use self-hypnosis. Everyone is different and each person has his or her own needs. Can self-hypnosis help you? Only you can answer that question. I frequently have patients tell me that they have been using this sort of self-suggestion for years but haven't called it self-hypnosis. They have learned the technique through trial and error. Counting sheep for insomnia might be thought of as a form of self-suggestion with the purpose of diverting attention from the stresses of the day. The highly susceptible person can learn self-hypnosis on his or her own. The less susceptible person will need some professional help. Whatever method you use, you will find it to useful in your everyday activities. My advice is to try it.

Many books are available to help you learn more about self-hypnosis. Some of the books are listed in the Suggested Reading section at the end of this book.

CHAPTER 7

Group Hypnosis

Remember that the hypnotist does not do anything to you; you do something for yourself. The hypnotist is the teacher and teaches you how to do it. Therefore, hypnosis can be used in a group setting just as can any other type of teaching. In group hypnosis the hypnotist offers suggestions to a group of people. It is up to each individual member of the group to decide whether or not to accept the suggestions and enter the trance state.

Reasons for group hypnosis vary depending on the

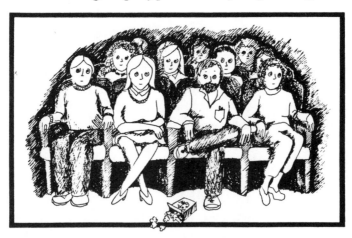

purpose of the group. Simple introduction to hypnosis as an interesting phenomenon might draw a group of people together. Another group of people may share a common problem, such as cigarette smoking. Still a third group may be pregnant women who are interested in learning relaxation techniques for childbirth. If group therapy does not produce the desired result, however, you should consider individual therapy.

I have used group hypnosis in workshops with 30 or more people interested in hypnotic techniques. In group hypnosis I give general suggestions for induction and deepening which would be acceptable for the average person. I explain the concept of hypnosis to the group and offer a simple induction technique and ideas for deepening. Then I provide positive suggestions regarding the purpose of the group and finally talk about the use of self-hypnosis for those interested in pursuing hypnosis for personal use.

If you were in the group, for instance, I would know nothing about your past experiences. I would not use the idea of descending in an elevator as a deepening suggestion since you may have a phobia about elevators. I would not suggest riding on a boat since you may have a problem with seasickness. I would not suggest anything which might cause an adverse reaction. Instead I would suggest activities such as walking through a sunken garden and seeing and smelling the flowers. I would suggest feeling the effects of the warm sun. I would suggest walking on a sandy beach or strolling through a wooded area. I might simply suggest that as I count slowly, you would gradually deepen the trance state. The higher or lower I count, the deeper the trance would be. I might be very permissive and suggest that you drift back in time to a very pleasant experience and relive the experience to its full extent. I might suggest that you go to a safe secure place in your mind. If you accepted these suggestions, you would enter a deeper trance state.

I remember a lecture at a national hypnosis convention during which the speaker asked everyone to enter the trance state by whatever means desired.

Since we were a group of experienced hypnotists, no further suggestions were necessary. He then suggested we take out a pencil and write automatically on a piece of paper the reason for coming to the conference. We were not to think of an answer, but simply let our hands write the response automatically. Lo and behold my hand began to write. I had no idea what I was writing. When he aroused us from the trance a little later, I found that I had written "Me." I assumed this to mean that I was attending the conference to find out more about my own mind. At least that seemed to be the reason as far as my subconscious mind was concerned.

I have been discussing one form of group hypnosis. The term can also apply to a group wherein everyone enters the trance state including the hypnotist. The members of the group then communicate while under the influence of their subconscious minds. Shirley Sanders, a teacher of hypnosis from North Carolina, has described this type of group hypnosis in a therapeutic setting. She calls this *mutual hypnosis* and uses it to help solve group problems. A troubled family with a drug-using teenager and an abusive father might find mutual hypnosis helpful for family interaction at a subconscious level. This type of therapy requires careful thought and the services of an expert hypnotist as well as an expert family counselor.

Group hypnosis has its limitations. The hypnotist must direct his or her suggestions to the average susceptibility of the members of the group. As a hypnotherapist I cannot address your personal problems if you are in a group. Therefore, I must go at a pace which is too fast for some and not fast enough for others. If you are not very susceptible to suggestion, you will be left behind. If you are very susceptible to suggestion, you will wish I would go faster. The advantage of individual therapy is that the trance can be paced to an individual's needs.

There are advantages to group therapy, too. Hypnotherapy is a form of psychotherapy, and the hypnotherapist charges fees on the basis of the time used. Group therapy allows many more people to benefit from the same amount of time, and individual fees are therefore generally less.

CHAPTER 8

Examples of The Use of Medical Hypnosis

Now that I have discussed medical hypnosis and the types of therapeutic suggestions that might be given, let's look at some specific examples to illustrate the various principles of medical hypnosis.

Case 1: M., a man in his 40's, came to me because of 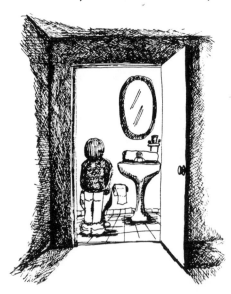 his phobia concerning restriction of his body. It was illustrated by his discomfort with the use of seat belts. He felt that a seat belt was too restrictive and became anxious when he wore one. His business required that he travel by airplane to give lectures at various locations in the United States. He carried a letter from his family doctor stating that he had the phobia and most airlines allowed him to fly with the seat belt applied only loosely. He realized that his fear was ridiculous, but he was unable to control it.

Unfortunately, he slipped on the ice one day and fractured his wrist. He had to wear a cast extending from his fingers to the middle part of the upper arm. As the plaster was being applied, he began to sweat. He said that he was afraid he might not be able to stand the constricted feeling of the plaster. The physician at the clinic treating the fracture laughed and said that he would get used to it like everyone else.

Later that evening he phoned the physician on call at the clinic stating that he simply couldn't stand the cast and that he was thinking of heading to the basement to hack it off with a hammer and saw. The physician realized that he was truly panicking over the cast. He advised M. to take a sedative that he happened to have in the house. M. took one, then two. Finally after he had taken four of them he was able to get to sleep. The next day he was still apprehensive about the cast, but thought he could live with it. When evening approached, he again began to panic. As he was starting for the basement to take the cast off, he realized that his panic was irrational and that he really needed the cast to allow the fracture to heal. He contacted yet another physician on call. Similar advice regarding sedatives was given. Finally he was able to sleep through the second night.

The following day, however, he decided he must do something about his fear and called me, knowing that I used medical hypnosis in my practice. I saw him that day and used hypnotic techniques to allow him to gain control over his phobia. I used a standard induction technique with non-specific deepening suggestions. While in a trance state, I suggested that he would be comfortable with the cast on his arm, that he would have a feeling of numbness in the arm and hand and that he would be able to function normally during the time that the cast was required. I repeated the hypnotherapy a week later to reinforce the ideas. I gave him a tape recording of the hypnotic suggestions.

I also taught him self-hypnosis so that he could continue to develop his tolerance to the cast as the days went by. He was able to wear the cast for the necessary four weeks without further difficulty. On only one occasion did he take one of his tranquilizers.

The hypnotherapy in this case required an hour on each of two visits and allowed the patient to be treated for a broken wrist in spite of his phobia of having any part of his body restricted. Although similar results could have been obtained with medication, he demonstrated that he required four times the normal amount for relief. Taking that amount of tranquilizer over a four week period would have been unwise. It would have caused him to be woozy much of the time and thus he would have been a danger to himself and others while driving. A psychiatrist or psychologist could have treated the phobia with psychotherapy, but such therapy takes a considerable length of time and the patient needed help without delay. His fracture healed well, and he was very pleased when the cast was finally removed.

Case 2: C had been a smoker for about 20 years. She smoked one to two packs of cigarettes a day. Her husband also smoked, and her teen-age children were picking up the habit. She was aware of the dangers of cigarette smoking. She had tried to quit smoking but was unable to stop for more than a day. She had enrolled in several classes to help her stop smoking, without success. She was well-motivated but simply unable to quit. She had heard of the use of hypnosis but felt that she could not be hypnotized and, even if she could, it wouldn't work for her. Anyway, what would her friends say if they knew she went to a hypnotist! She finally decided to seek help from me without telling anyone, not even her husband. She was a satisfactory hypnotic subject and entered the trance state without any real problem. I gave her several suggestions about being a nonsmoker. I then advised her to practice self-hypnosis three to four times a day and to enjoy the new lifestyle of a nonsmoker. Finally I gave her a tape recording of the trance so that she could use it if her self-hypnosis wasn't as successful as she desired. One visit of one hour sufficed, and a year later, she was still a nonsmoker. By then, of course, she had told her husband and friends how she had kicked the habit.

This case illustrates another medical use of hypnosis. Cigarette smoking is one of the major causes of death in the United States. It is now considered to be a true addiction which is very difficult to control. I have seen people with advanced lung disease continue to smoke in spite of the knowledge that they are literally killing themselves. I would be remiss to suggest to you that hypnosis is always successful for people wishing to become nonsmokers. The success rate varies from one therapist to another, but with proper motivation and persistence, it is successful often enough to be considered a useful form of therapy. Further sessions are sometimes necessary for patients who are less susceptible, or are unable to succeed with a single visit. Other habits such as fingernail biting and bed wetting can often be treated with hypnosis as well.

The case of C illustrates another common misunderstanding. Although she felt she couldn't be hypnotized, she was able to benefit from the technique.

Case 3: L, a terminal cancer patient, was in the hospital suffering from severe pain throughout most of her body. She was on many pain medications and lying in a special bed that allowed even distribution of pressure on her back and legs. She was not expected to live more than a few weeks and wished desperately to be allowed to go home for her last days. Her doctors, however, knew that she would need hospital care unless they were able to control her pain. I saw her for one visit, and, though she was not very responsive due to the effects of her medications, I was able to give her suggestions about re-experiencing in her mind pleasurable past events. She chose to recall days spent working in her garden. I knew that I had helped her when I was informed later that she was more comfortable and that she was talking about the various colors of the flowers in her imaginary garden. She returned home and died a few weeks later.

This case illustrates how patients with pain, even if under the influence of narcotics, can be helped with hypnotherapy. Since I was only able to see her on one brief occasion, I wasn't able to pursue other hypnotherapeutic possibilities for her.

Case 4: J., a boy of about 7, wet his bed nearly every night. He was a perfectly normal boy in every other way. His parents were very supportive as he tried to stop wetting the bed, but his mother was tired of changing his bed every day. She aroused him an hour or two after he went to bed, but frequently he was already wet at that time. She tried having him change his own sheets and even threatened him with loss of privileges, but nothing worked. She had heard of a friend's child being helped with hypnosis so she brought him to me.

J. was rather shy, but I talked to him about some of the things he liked to do and gradually gained his confidence. I asked him if he would like to play a game with me, and he agreed. Since children are very imaginative, they rapidly enter the trance state. He responded to the suggestion that he imagine watching his favorite television program. He easily became involved with the program, and I implanted in his sub-conscious mind several suggestions. I suggested that he awaken during the night when he had the urge to urinate, go to the bathroom, urinate in the toilet, go back to a warm dry bed, and sleep soundly the rest of the night. I taught him how to give himself the suggestions and practice self-hypnosis. He didn't stop wetting the bed all at once, but after several weeks the bed was wet less often and finally it was wet only on rare occasions. He was proud to have gained control of his problem.

Enuresis, or bed wetting, is a very common problem, especially with boys. There are several means of dealing with it. Medications are useful as well as the "bell and pad" method, behavioral therapy, and superficial psychotherapy. The bell and pad method requires a pad to be placed under the patient. When it becomes wet, it causes a bell to ring and the patient to awaken. Hypnosis is frequently helpful as a primary method of treatment or when other methods have failed.

Although hypnotherapy isn't always successful, it has helped many patients with a wide variety of problems. The patient's motivation and his or her willingness to use a tape of their session with the therapist to re-experience the hypnotic suggestions or to practice self-hypnosis several times daily are prime factors in success. In the following chapters, I will discuss in more detail how hypnotherapy can be used to treat specific problems.

CHAPTER 9

Hypnosis to Stop Smoking

Let's assume that you are a woman who wants hypnotherapy to help you quit cigarette smoking. Certainly everything you have read about smoking confirms that it is bad for your health and also for the health of your children since they breathe in your sec-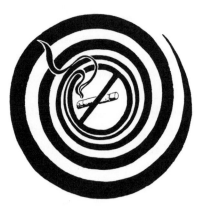ond hand smoke. You have tried to quit many times, only to revert to the habit when your willpower was down and a friend offered you a cigarette. Remember the Law of Reversed Effect that I discussed in Chapter 5. It is very difficult to become a nonsmoker and very easy after being a nonsmoker for a while to have "just one." "Just one" usually leads you into full-time smoking again.

Let's also assume that you have obtained my name as a medical hypnotist and that you call for an appointment. An appointment is set up, and you spend the next few days trying to decide if you really want to keep it or not. You finally decide to go through with it, even though you aren't really sure that you want to quit smoking.

At the office, you nervously wait to see the doctor. Will he be scary? Will he have a long pointed beard? Will he look different from other people? Heavens, maybe you had better get out while the getting is good! The waiting room seems pleasant enough. There is that old lady with her husband waiting to be seen. There are those little children playing in the children's corner. Oh, well, you guess that you will see it through.

When I come out to greet you, you decide that I'm really not an ogre. I seem friendly enough, and although I have a beard, it isn't pointed. I don't have the air of hocus-pocus about me. Things seem to be settling down a bit. You accept my greeting, participate in small talk about the weather, and become more at ease. I take you to a comfortable examining room with a reclining chair but instead you choose an upright chair. You think, "He's going to have a problem getting me in that recliner."

I ask you a few questions about your smoking habit. When did you start? How many cigarettes do you smoke in a typical day? What type do you smoke? Does anyone else in the family smoke? Can you smoke at work? Do your children object to your smoking? Does your husband? Why have you decided to be a nonsmoker at this particular time? Next, I ask you what you know about hypnosis. You tell me that you have seen it on TV, but otherwise you don't know anything about it. I spend about half an hour describing the trance, the trance state and hypnosis. I explain how a person responds to suggestion naturally and explain the concept of daydreaming as a form of trance. I discuss briefly the idea of alternate states of consciousness and stress the naturalness of the hypnotic trance. I also explain that my suggestions will be positive and will describe nonsmoking as the desired result. Since I feel that "quitting" anything is a negative idea, I prefer not using that word. Instead I stress the positive reasons for becoming and remaining a nonsmoker. You ask some questions and I answer

them at what I perceive to be your level of understanding. I stress that I cannot promise success and
that your motivation in becoming a nonsmoker is
much more important than any technique I may use
or your level of hypnotizability.

Next, I suggest that we use a test trance to determine what types of suggestions you respond to best. I
suggest that the recliner might be more comfortable,
and I turn down the lights so that you are not distract-
ed by the bright lights. I mention that you will be able
to hear outside noises such as a truck or airplane, or
perhaps the paging system, but that those noises have
nothing to do with your treatment, so they can be dis-
regarded. I choose an induction that is suitable for the
moment. As an example I might ask you to roll your
eyes up to the top of your head, and while relaxing,
gently close your eyelids over your upturned eyes. I
use the same basic test trance deepening suggestions
described in the Chapter 4.

Following your arousal from the test trance you
might tell me that you responded well to relaxation
and age regression suggestions. I give you a chance to
ask questions, and I explain what I have done. Since
you are very relaxed and seem ready for therapeutic
suggestions, I hook up the tape recorder and typically
proceed as follows.

Roll your eyes up now and gently let your eyelids
close. Go down, down, down, down into a very relaxed state.....See the kitten lying in the sun. Feel your
body, like the kitten, become completely relaxed and
at ease.....Drift back in time to a wonderful experience...Relive that experience. See it...Feel it...Taste
it...Enjoy it.....

Now continue to feel relaxed and at ease. Continue to enjoy the experience. Continue to pay attention
to me and ignore all outside sounds and thoughts......

Consider the reasons why you are here. Consider your life as a nonsmoker...You are a nonsmoker now because you have decided to be a nonsmoker. It's simply a matter of remaining a nonsmoker... Walk down a path with me and come to a signpost. One sign says "smoker" and the other says "nonsmoker." Follow the sign that says "nonsmoker" and join all of the other nonsmokers...... Think of the many advantages of being a nonsmoker. The money saved. The health benefits. The health of your children. The ability to taste things better and to smell things better. The reduced risk of fire.....You only have one body in this life, and smoking is a danger to that body. You owe your body respect and protection. Let this idea sink deeply into your subconscious: "I am now a nonsmoker and I will remain a nonsmoker." .....Allow your mind to drift deeper and deeper.....

I will explain a little bit about self-hypnosis. I want you to practice either with this tape or with self-hypnosis at least four times a day. Self-hypnosis is pretty much the same as this trance, except I will not be there teaching you. Your own conscious mind will be instructing your subconscious. It is much like talking to yourself, but it is a more active process whereby your conscious mind teaches your subconscious mind what you want it to do.....Simply find a comfortable place to relax...Roll your eyes upward and let them close...Think about relaxation. Just let yourself go.....Go back in time to the pleasant experience. Your conscious mind will be subdued, but it will continue to be in control... Give yourself positive suggestions about your being a nonsmoker. Suggest that the positive suggestions will continue and persist even when you are no longer in the trance state. Suggest that the next time you enter a trance it will be faster, easier and at a deeper level.....When you are ready to arouse from this trance and from your own trances at home, say to yourself, "I will arouse now realizing that the effects of the suggestions will persist and I will be able to enter the trance easily and rapidly next time." Then, taking your time, simply open your eyes and you won't be in the trance any more.

When you actually arouse from the trance, you feel very relaxed and at ease. You are confident that you are now and will continue to be a nonsmoker. You plan to practice hypnosis four times a day, and by thus barring the temptation of taking another cigarette, you are cured of your habit. You take the tape after my reassurance that I will be available if you have any further questions or need further therapy.

Although this verbalization of the hypnotic suggestions is brief, I allow time for deepening suggestions to take effect and repeat many of the therapeutic phrases for greater effect. No two therapeutic trances are the same because no two people are the same. The time of the actual hypnotic trance ranges from 5 to 20 minutes. The therapist varies his or her verbalization depending on the situation, while staying within the basic framework of the four steps for therapeutic hypnosis.

CHAPTER 10

Hypnosis for a Pregnant Patient

Nancy and her husband had wanted to start a family for a number of months and had not been using birth control. When she missed a menstrual period, she excitedly came to see me, her family physician,

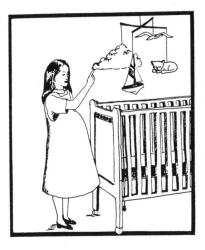

for confirmation of a pregnancy. In the excitement of the visit she neglected to tell me that she had been having some morning sickness, but on a later visit she related that she was feeling quite miserable. She also confessed to having a deep-seated fear of delivery because her mother and an aunt had told her some horror stories about their own pregnancies and deliveries.

Nancy was not a unique patient. Many young women have *hyperemesis gravidarum*, or vomiting during pregnancy. Also, many young women fear the delivery experience despite many newer approaches to delivery such as Lamaze techniques, natural childbirth, and various anesthetics. Simple reassurance seldom takes care of such a problem. I suggested the use of hypnosis to help Nancy have a more comfortable pregnancy and childbirth. First, I was attentive to the many purely medical aspects of her pregnancy and ordered the necessary laboratory tests. I gave Nancy educational materials and reviewed them with her. I encouraged the office personnel, particularly the office nurses, to become involved with her care so that she would feel comfortable calling them to ask questions. We needed to work as a team. After seeing to all of these things, I discussed with her how hypnosis might be helpful in her case.

After dealing with the regular medical aspects of her pregnancy, I set up an appointment for training in hypnosis. During that hour-long visit I explained what hypnosis is and what it is not. I was careful to clarify and dispel the myths surrounding hypnosis. I explained many of the concepts described in this book. She was comfortable with the ideas and wished to proceed. To determine how susceptible she was to entering the hypnotic trance state and to what types of suggestions she would best respond, I gave her the simple hypnotic test.

Nancy was a good subject, about a 3.5 on a scale of 1 to 5, in which a person classified as a 1 is poorly hypnotizable and a person classified as a 5 is considered to be an excellent subject. Since Nancy was slightly above average, she should do well if she were willing to practice the techniques. She responded well to relaxation, visual suggestions and age regression, but did not respond well to hearing or feeling suggestions. We decided to work on the problem of morning sickness first. At later visits we would focus on her anxiety regarding giving birth. We discussed ways to ease her labor and delivery. We didn't plan to stop there, however, because hypnosis is also useful in preparing her for the days and weeks after delivery.

There are many theories about the cause of nausea during pregnancy. Some doctors feel that it is psychological. Others feel that it is not just in the mind. I see it as a combination of the two. Some women require only a small amount of positive suggestion to cure the problem. These women tend to be convinced that they will have the problem. Perhaps their mothers or sisters suffered from it. The problem in these cases seems to be primarily psychological. On the other hand, I have treated some women who did not respond to hypnosis. Either they simply did not respond to the suggestions or their problem was caused by the body and not the mind.

A condensed version of my approach in Nancy's case follows. I spoke in a slow, distinct, rather monotonous voice. The induction and deepening suggestions were similar to those used in Chapter 9.

> Let your mind and body become completely relaxed. Be aware that this wonderful sense of peace and relaxation will continue with you for the rest of the day, even when you aren't in the trance anymore. Enjoy eating food and drinking water, juices, and other liquids. Let these nourishing foods settle easily in your stomach so that both you and your baby can benefit from them. There is no need for being uncomfortable as your pregnancy progresses. Enjoy the feelings as the little child grows. Ease, comfort, relaxation, tranquillity, and serenity will continue to be a part of your life. I suggest that you will continue to be free of discomfort even after you come out of the trance and that you will be able to eat and drink comfortably the rest of today, tonight, and tomorrow, continuing into the future. I suggest that the next time you use hypnosis, you will be able to enter the trance state faster and easier and deeper. The act of rolling your eyes to the top of your head will act as a cue to help enter

the trance state. I also suggest that you use self-hypnosis or use a tape of this session at least four times each day. I will now turn this trance over to you so that you can continue to think about these ideas and transfer them to your subconscious mind where they will be most helpful. When you are ready to come out of the trance state, you can do so by simply deciding to open your eyes.

I made a cassette tape of the session and gave it to her. I urged her to use it four times a day just as I might a drug prescription. We then set up another appointment in a week.

At the next visit, we discussed her progress. She had been diligent in practicing and had been less nauseated. I encouraged her to continue practicing her hypnosis four times a day. She mentioned that she was still working and found it difficult to get in the noon session. I acknowledged that it is sometimes difficult to comply but encouraged her to practice as many times a day as possible under her circumstances.

During the next visit, I repeated the therapeutic trance and added suggestions that Nancy should begin preparing for the delivery. I stressed the importance of relaxation as part of the delivery process, both for her comfort and for the comfort of the baby. Tight and tense muscles make relaxation of the birth canal more difficult, thereby lengthening the delivery process. Learning to relax the muscles of the pelvis, both consciously and subconsciously through the hypnotic process, would allow her to have an easier and more rapid delivery. After the hypnosis session, I began teaching her about the nature of labor and delivery.

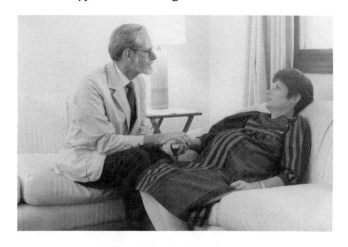

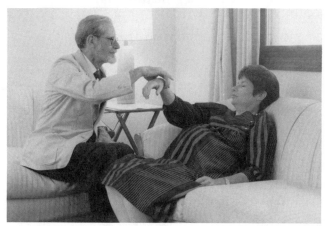

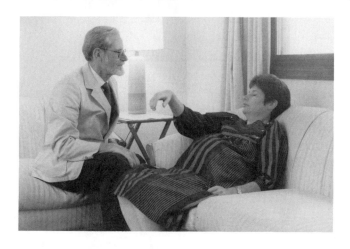

A example of hypnotic induction in a pregnant patient

I urged to her to attend birthing classes with her husband and to read books on the subject. I urged her to continue practicing self-hypnosis and gave her the cassette tape of that visit's hypnosis session.

Later visits followed a similar routine. I included hypnosis training during six of these visits. I introduced ideas for the management of discomfort including dissociation, distraction, deep relaxation techniques, and time distortion. I also introduced the concept of bonding with the baby and offered suggestions to assist her in the enjoyment of nursing the baby. I mentioned the possibility of the commonly experienced mild depression frequently present after the birth of the baby. As Nancy's pregnancy progressed, she continued to practice several times a day, and nausea was no longer a problem. Nancy had her baby several days early. She used self-hypnosis through much of her labor and required only one small injection of an anesthetic for discomfort. She was awake and beaming immediately after the birth of a beautiful baby girl. Her husband was there to support her and her medical course after the delivery was uneventful.

CHAPTER 11

Hypnosis for Sexual Problems

Physical conditions may cause sexual problems. A woman with a tight, narrow vagina might experience 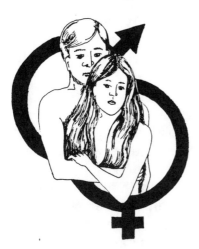 discomfort with penetration of the penis. She might carry the virus causing herpes simplex, which causes pain. A man might have inability to achieve an erection due to poor blood flow to the penis from arteriosclerosis, particularly if he has diabetes mellitus. He might have pain with erection due to Peyronie's disease, which is a condition manifested by fibrous tissue within the penis itself.

Psychological factors, however, are often responsible for sexual problems. For example, fear of inadequate performance accounts for most cases of *preorgasmia*, formerly called *frigidity* in women and *impotence* in men. (The term frigidity is seldom used now because it implies the permanent loss of the ability for a woman to experience orgasm. The term preorgasmia indicates that orgasm can be achieved with proper training.) Long-established psychological problems may require prolonged therapy. Sexual counselors, couples' counselors, practitioners of behavior modification, psychologists, and psychiatrists are trained to treat patients with sexual problems.

The hypnotherapist, however, has a great deal to offer. Many sexual problems respond well to hypnotherapy. Hypnosis is particularly useful for the person who is unable to relax and enjoy his or her sexual functioning.

Suggestions given during hypnotherapy would include those that would help the patient to relax, improve his or her self-confidence, and anticipate the sex act with confidence in the ability to succeed. Relaxation techniques are useful in these instances because relaxation during sexual activity is more likely to result in a successful sexual experience.

A woman can be taught to respond to sexual stimulation by various techniques described in manuals on sexuality. Hypnosis can also play a part by allowing her to be able to accept such techniques without biases learned in her youth. Positive suggestions are always in order when we deal with the subconscious, and with pre-orgasmia the primary goal of hypnotherapy is to instill confidence. The woman is instructed to relax during intercourse and to teach her partner how to best stimulate her to reach orgasm. Kinsey revealed through his experiments that women take longer to reach orgasm than men. Unfortunately, most men are not aware of this. Proper instruction for both partners will help a woman achieve orgasm. Hypnotic suggestion provides a woman with a method of enhancing her relaxation and self-confidence.

Pain during intercourse is called *dyspareunia*. It is a significant problem for many women. Possible physical causes of dyspareunia must be ruled out before psychological methods are used. A current or an old infection in the pelvic organs, pre-menstrual tension, and injury to the vagina from childbirth or surgery can result in pain. Fear of intercourse may lead to spasm and tightening of the muscles and cause pain. *Vaginismus* is a condition in which the muscles of the pelvis are so much in spasm that normal intercourse is impossible. Dyspareunia can sometimes be treated with a change in sexual technique or position so that the area of pain can be avoided. Anesthetic creams are useful if the cause of pain is localized to the vaginal opening or the vagina itself. Various forms of psychotherapy can be helpful for this problem. Relaxation techniques, biofeedback, and hypnotic suggestions have been found to be useful for these women.

For a man, *premature ejaculation* is an example of a condition which frequently responds to hypnotherapy. Premature ejaculation refers to male orgasm before a couple wishes it to happen, often immediately upon insertion of the penis into the vagina. This does not allow for a prolonged, leisurely form of intercourse. Various forms of treatment for this condition have been described in the literature on sexuality. An example is the *pinch technique* described by Kinsey. Orgasm is averted by pinching the area beneath the head of the penis. A more permanent means of postponing orgasm is by the use of hypnotic suggestion. During the hypnotic trance, suggestions are given that the patient will be able to postpone his orgasm by being more relaxed and at ease. Suggestions of attention diversion are also helpful. These suggestions are incorporated into post-hypnotic suggestions so that the patient can respond to them when he is not actually in the trance state. Suggestions of lessening of sensation in the penis are also useful for some men. This will allow more active intercourse without orgasm before it is desired. The techniques used for decreasing sensation will be discussed in the chapter on pain control.

Impotence is a man's inability to achieve or sustain an erection. Dr. Harold Crasileneck, a well-respected hypnotherapist from Dallas, Texas, uses a novel approach for treating impotence. He suggests that the firmness of an erection is similar to *catalepsy* of the patient's arm. Catalepsy means the inability to move a joint. As an example, hypnotists might suggest during a trance state that the arm of a subject will become straight and firm and that it will be immovable no matter how hard he or she may try to bend it. The subject is usually unable to do so, and the association is made that the firmness of the arm can be transferred to the penis. This technique may seem ridiculous, but it is frequently successful. Remember that the subconscious part of the mind cannot think and what might seem ridiculous to the conscious mind is frequently effective when acted on by the subconscious. Just giving the patient the idea that something can be done about impotence may be enough to relieve the problem.

The following paraphrase of a case history will help illustrate how hypnosis was used for a sexual problem:

Mrs. R., a 26-year-old factory worker, had been married for 8 years. Her husband, aged 31 years, was a sales manager. She was referred for sexual counseling by a psychiatrist with "not having consummated her marriage" as the presenting problem. She had seen 11 doctors for the problem over the eight years of her marriage. Treatments had included drugs designed to alter the mind and attempted psychoanalysis. Mrs. R. had decided to seek help yet again because of her strong desire to have a child. She had had a disturbed relationship with both her parents. She was tearful in discussing her mother who had died six weeks prior to her marriage. She had great misgivings toward the medical and allied professions resulting from a series of injections she received at two years of age. She had received minimal sexual education and even that had carried negative implications.

She had no history of major psychiatric illnesses. During her first visit, significant information included a high level of anxiety, failure to accept her own sexuality, and the fear of vaginal penetration which had generalized to fear of other penetrations such as tongue kissing or enema insertion. She was, however, able to participate in a form of mutual masturbation with her husband when fully clothed and without direct genital play. She was generally inhibited in interpersonal relationships and reticent in expressing any hostility directly.

Mr. R. was present at the initial interview. He had never had intercourse but had no difficulty with erection or ejaculation during masturbation. He seemed optimistic and relaxed about the outcome, claiming that there was always a way around problems. Mrs. R. was seen in individual therapy over the next 16 months. Her husband was seen intermittently during this time.

Autogenic techniques, a form of hypnosis, were taught to Mrs. R. in order to reduce her general level of anxiety. The use of hypnosis seemed to accelerate the positive relationship between her and her therapist. As her family conflicts were explored, hypnosis was utilized to systematically desensitize Mrs. R. to her own genitalia.

Following desensitization to looking at her genitalia, Mrs. R. was for the first time able to shower with her husband. From time to time she would describe rape fantasies and dreams and comment that she wished her husband would be more assertive. She was successively desensitized to touching the genitalia and vaginal penetration with one, two, and three fingers and tampons. At this stage Mrs. R. had an argument with her husband over an inconsequential matter and withdrew herself from all contact with him for the ensuing month.

Psychotherapy helped her to admit and cope with her anger and resentment toward her parents. In the therapeutic encounter as in her marriage, she tended to take the role of a child being helped by a parent. Therapy was directed at making her aware of this and encouraging her to assume adulthood. She was also encouraged to explore and admit to her sexual thoughts and fantasies. Some six months after weekly therapy sessions began, Mrs. R. initiated sexual intercourse and the marriage was consummated. The consummation was preceded by a dream in which she saw the therapist and the therapist's husband walking hand in hand past her childhood home. She was cross because they appeared happy and she felt shut off. Interestingly, Mrs. R.'s husband had some initial problems achieving an erection in the first few weeks after penetration.

Sexual intercourse, an almost daily phenomenon from then on, proceeded from being purely mechanical for Mrs. R. to an act that gradually allowed pleasure. Five weeks after consummation, she requested a vaginal examination which was accomplished with no evidence of anxiety. The couple both reported that although they had a good relationship prior to therapy, it had markedly improved in quality since it began.

Eight months after therapy commenced, Mrs. R. became pregnant. The prospect of motherhood revived her own early experience of being mothered. She became convinced that her mother, until now described as overprotective, had in fact rejected her. Discussions with an aunt confirmed her suspicions that she had been unplanned, unwanted, and rejected by her mother until the age of two. After she became seriously ill, her mother had suddenly accepted her and prevented other family members from relating with her. Although Mrs. R. was at last able to understand her ambivalence toward her parents, she became anxious about her own ability to mother. She feared that she also would either reject or smother her own infant. She also had many concerns relating to pregnancy, childbirth and hospitalization. She continued to be seen by her therapist on a weekly basis throughout her pregnancy. Hypnosis was used to help desensitize her to the concept of labor and hospitalization. The hypnotic techniques she had been taught were now emphasized as a coping strategy for the anxiety and panic feeling she feared. Hypnotherapy sessions were also used to increase her self-esteem and confidence in her ability to mother.

Seventeen months after therapy began, Mrs. R. had healthy twin boys, four weeks prematurely. She required no analgesia during the first stage of labor but had an anesthetic for a forceps delivery of the first twin and breech delivery of the second.

Both babies required incubator care during the days following birth. Mrs. R. became tearful and increasingly distressed. Hypnosis was used to help her express her fears that her poor mothering had resulted in her babies' present ill health. Intervention with nursing and pediatric staff resulted in Mrs. R. being given increased access to the babies and information about their progress. Bonding proceeded uneventfully. Eighteen months later, she was coping well with both babies and her marriage.*

---

*(Condensed from Lorraine Dennerstein, "Hypnosis and Psychosexual Dysfunction" in Handbook of Hypnosis and Psychosomatic Medicine, Graham D. Burrows and Lorraine Dennerstein, eds. Elsevier/North-Holland Biomedical Press, 1980, 354.)

Sexual activity is a normal and necessary part of human existence. Without it, humanity would have become extinct long ago. It is an enjoyable physiological function. Unfortunately, it also leads to emotional turmoil. Moral, legal and religious aspects of sexual activity are significant factors. Diseases which can be contracted through intercourse have become a life and death matter. Emotional response to sexual activity leads to problems. Since sex is here to stay we frequently need therapeutic measures for sexual problems. Hypnotherapy is a useful form of therapy for this purpose.

CHAPTER 12

Hypnosis for Patients in Pain

Pain presents an enormous problem for our society. It has been estimated that five billion dollars is spent annually on medical costs, drugs, and lost work because of chronic pain. It would be wonderful if hypnosis were truly a wonder drug. Unfortunately, in dealing with the human mind, nothing is perfect. Although wonderful things can be accomplished in many patients, there are people who do not respond

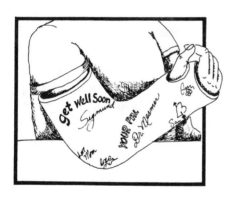

to hypnotherapy for pain problems. I have seen patients respond beautifully to hypnotic suggestions and also those who have not benefited from it at all. Unfortunately, some of those who did not respond actually felt worse since yet another type of treatment had been tried and had failed. I feel that it is worth the effort, however, since the successful patient has much to gain.

We all know what pain feels like, but it is difficult to define. Simply put, pain is the perception of something gone wrong and that whatever has gone wrong hurts. Pain is an essential bodily function; it is the major protective device that keeps us from injuring ourselves. Once the cause of a pain is known, something can be done about relieving it and attending to the cause. When pain persists after it is no longer needed for our protection, however, it becomes a problem, and medical science is called upon to deal with it.

The experience of feeling pain can be divided into two basic parts. First, there is the reflex response to the injury. This is the protective mechanism that causes us to withdraw a burned finger from the stove or a punctured foot from a nail. Second, there is the suffering. Suffering involves much more than physical pain. It includes the worry about loss of work due to the injury or painful disease. It might include postponing a much anticipated vacation since you can't swim in the Caribbean with a cast on a broken arm. It might include concerns about facing friends after stupidly falling off a ladder. It includes all of the factors involved in an injury or disease excepting the physical pain. Actually, this aspect of pain may be much harder to endure than the physical pain. A dog experiences pain when struck by a car. He doesn't have the mental capacity, however, to endure the many other aspects of suffering that humans do. Considering pain as a medical and social problem necessitates dividing it into several stages. Although many classifications exist, I prefer the following classification system which divides pain into four basic categories or stages: acute pain, subacute pain, chronic pain and subchronic pain. Hypnosis can be useful in each of the stages, but different hypnotherapeutic approaches are needed for each stage.

Acute Pain

Acute pain lasts up to two months, and during this time the patient expects to recover completely. Injury causes most types of acute pain. Various psychological tests has been found useful for a better understanding of how the mind reacts to the various stages of pain. The Minnesota Multiphasic Personality Inventory (MMPI) is such a test. It has many applications in the evaluation of patients such as the findings of depression, hypochondria, or hysteria. It has little application in acute pain, but when used experimentally, the scores have been found to be no different whether the patient is in acute pain or not.

Acute pain, being of relatively short duration, does not require more from the physician than reassurance that routine medical forms of treatment will take care of the problem. Hypnosis, however, can be useful as a technique to help relieve acute pain. At the time of an injury, for example, a patient is highly motivated to do something about the discomfort. He or she can readily enter the trance state by following suggestions of relaxation and suggestions which are designed to divert attention.

Hypnosis is especially useful in children over the age of five when they are capable of concentrated attention. I usually ask a child with a broken arm, for example, what his or her favorite TV show might be. This is an unexpected question, and attention is briefly diverted from the broken arm. The patient may say "Sesame Street." I say, "Would you like to watch Sesame Street now?" The child looks around for a TV set but doesn't see one, so I say, "Just close your eyes and see the TV set at home." This becomes a game and children are good at games. After a little while, I add, "Do you see it?" Usually there is a nod of affirmation. I then say, "Why don't you keep watching Sesame Street and I'll put some numbing medicine on your arm so it won't hurt." While children enter trances rapidly, they arouse just as rapidly, so I have to keep offering suggestions regarding the TV show that is being watched. I can obtain the x-rays, inject the fracture site if necessary, and put on the cast while the child is watching Sesame Street within his or her own mind. When the treatment is all finished, I suggest that the program is done and that the eyes can open again. I have talked the child into entering a trance state and have used it to divert attention away from my caring for the broken arm. I have used the simple technique of diversion of attention.

Most adults lack the imagination to follow the approach used with a child. They know better than to go along with something as silly as closing their eyes and watching TV. I must accept their feelings of skepticism. If the adult is in acute pain and is suggestible, however, and is willing to use hypnosis, it is worth the time that it takes for a more formal hypnotic induction. Since the adult tends to need more explanation, I must take the time to prepare him or her for hypnosis. A person might enjoy reliving a fishing trip through the hypnotic trance state as I treat his injury, or might choose any of a number of pastimes during the treatment. Pain is subjective. By diverting attention away from it, I have helped reduce the suffering which accompanies the physical pain.

Subacute Pain

Subacute pain may follow acute pain and lasts from two to about six months. A patient who still hurts after several months wonders why. There are many reasons for pain to persist, but the patient expects it to be gone by then. If the MMPI is given to a patient with subacute pain his or her answers may suggest hypochondria and/or hysteria. Such answers indicate only minor changes rather than serious changes in the personality.

The use of hypnosis for subacute pain depends on the situation at the time. Diversion of attention no longer suffices since the pain itself has become a source of worry. The post hypnotic suggestion of a feeling of numbness in the painful area might help the patient be free of pain for extended periods of time. Suggestions that are used for chronic pain might be useful at this stage, but patients seldom seek help from a hypnotherapist at the subacute stage of pain.

Chronic Pain

With chronic pain, which has usually lasted for more than six months, some basic changes in the personality might occur. The patient gradually realizes that the pain may never go away. He or she has visited a number of doctors representing various specialties for pain relief, to no avail. The person with the pain has probably been told, "You will just have to learn to live with it." Friends and relatives tend to ignore the patient's complaints. Marked depression, triggered by the realization that the pain may be permanent, is common during this stage. There may be sleep disturbances, loss of self-esteem, feelings of guilt, sexual problems, and thoughts of suicide.

If the MMPI is given to a patient with chronic pain, the scores may reveal evidence of hypochondria, hysteria, and depression. These are more profound changes in the personality. Patients with such scores are sometimes unjustly labeled as "pain prone," "low back losers," or "pain neurotics."

Causes of chronic pain include such diverse problems as myofascial syndrome, diabetic foot pain, cancer pain, phantom limb pain after an amputation, low back pain following a lumbar disk injury which has not responded to surgery, and migraine headaches. Myofascial syndrome can be the source of chronic pain. It is a poorly understood condition in which there is localized pain in muscle groups, particularly in the region of the upper back and neck. The condition tends to respond poorly to medications and does not have a surgical cure. Diabetic neuropathy is a condition which may occur in patients with diabetes mellitus where there is burning pain in the hands and feet. Again it responds poorly to medication and there is little that can be done in the way of surgery.

Patients with chronic pain present a much greater challenge to the medical community than patients with acute or subacute pain. The suffering aspect of pain becomes significant since work is lost, vacations aren't enjoyable, and just living becomes a burden. The onset of depression makes the pain much harder to bear.

Treatment requires a team approach. The team might include physical therapists, psychologists, physicians, nurses, pharmacologists, surgeons, social workers, and family therapists. The hypnotist can be helpful as part of the team. He or she can deal directly with the patient's subconscious mind, offering suggestions to bolster the patient's own recovery potential.

The primary duty of the hypnotist is to offer the patient some personal control over the problem. When we enter the medical arena as patients for whatever reason, we lose much of our control. This is especially true in an intensive care unit. We are hooked up to a myriad of tubes, wires, and electronic gadgets and can hardly move from side to side. We may not even be able to talk if there is a tube in the throat. The doctors, nurses, respiratory therapists, physical therapists, etc., are all there to help us, but we have almost no personal control over the situation. When we are in chronic pain, we feel that we have lost control over our bodies. We can only undergo the surgery that is suggested, take the pills that are prescribed, and go in for physical therapy that itself may be painful. How can we regain some feeling of control?

A person who has learned to use self-hypnosis has learned a degree of self-control. As a hypnotist, my first task is to give patients this feeling of control. As a patient I can always, no matter what the circumstance, leave the conscious world and enter the hypnotic trance state. No matter whether I am in pain, bored with what is going on, trying to get to sleep, or feeling anxious about something, I can divert my attention from the action around me. I can determine how I wish to feel about an event. I can control my thoughts, allowing me to enjoy a pleasant experience. I can control my muscular tenseness, secretions, sensations and sense of time. In other words, I have gained an extremely important feeling of control over my destiny.

As a hypnotherapist, I can also suggest other options for pain control. Patients may learn to turn down the intensity of the pain as though they were turning down the temperature control on the furnace. They can learn to divert their attention from the pain to an enjoyable thought or activity. They can learn to change the sensation of pain to that of itching, numbness or pressure, and they can learn to distort the concept of time so that it seems to go faster during times of pain. They can learn to build their egos to better handle the pain. They can take time-outs in which there is relief from the pain, perhaps mentally enjoying a favorite hobby or pastime.

Subchronic Pain

The stage of pain which I term *subchronic* some-times follows chronic pain. At this time the person with the pain has accepted it and no longer seeks a cure. He or she lives a perhaps limited but satisfacto-ry life. This stage is the therapeutic goal for the pa-tient with chronic pain. It can begin at any time in the process, but requires the patient's cooperation in working toward the goal of acceptance and accommo-dation. The patient realizes that the pain will proba-bly persist no matter what medical or surgical inter-vention is used. He or she begins to function more normally in spite of the pain. Symptoms of depression decline or disappear. When an MMPI is given to the patient at this stage, the scores on the depression scale usually approach normal, although the hypochondria and hysteria scores are generally elevated.

Two case examples from the medical literature may help explain how hypnosis can be of use for patients with chronic pain.

Patient 1: A 42 year old woman suffered a five-year history of trigeminal neuralgia (a very painful condition involving one of the nerves of the face). Unsuccessful surgical intervention and many phar-macological regimens were tried. Pain was consid-ered to be very severe, rated at "8" and "10" (on a 0 to 10 scale of severity). The pain frequently caused her to miss work. As a last resort, her neurosurgeon referred her to the pain clinic for evaluation. The patient was estimated to be in the midrange of hypnotic capacity. After undergoing a thorough evaluation, the patient was taught to use a substituted sensation for the pain. She was able to enter into a trance state and allowed the pain to be experienced in minimal amounts by condensing her experience and by substituting another sensation (tingling).

Although initially the patient did not receive the results she had anticipated, with patience and encouragement (in about five sessions) she was able to apply successful hypnotic intervention which helped her to control her pain and then minimize the discomfort. Not only was she able to control pain while it was occurring, but her anticipation of the pain was also decreased.

Patient 2: A 30 year old woman had a five year history of low back pain and had undergone six unsuccessful surgical procedures. Pharmacological agents were causing further complications for the patient. She complained of almost continuous pain and had to withdraw from graduate school.

Following appropriate evaluation, it was determined that the patient had a mid to high hypnotic capacity. She was able to remove the pain directly by getting an analgesic response. The strategy developed was based on her previous experiences in obtaining this similar response with pharmacological and anesthetic blocks. She was able to experience coldness and as such was able to reinforce herself and thus remove the pain. Following her successful hypnotic intervention, she was eventually able to return to graduate school, write her dissertation and obtain her graduate degree.*

---

*Harold J. Wain, Ph.D., *Hypnosis in the Treatment of Chronic Pain: Clinical Hypnosis in Medicine*, Harold J. Wain, Ph.D., Yearbook Medical Publishers, Chicago, 1980, p. 7.

CHAPTER 13

Multiple Personality Disorder

Several popular novels have been written about persons with *multiple personality disorder*. It is a serious mental condition in which an individual has several distinct personalities. It has been defined by Taylor and Martin as "two or more personalities (in one body) each of which is so well developed and integrated as to have a relatively coordinated, rich, unified, and stable life of its own." Each personality is unaware of the existence of the others. There is a central all-knowing part of the mind of these persons, however, which can be used in therapy.

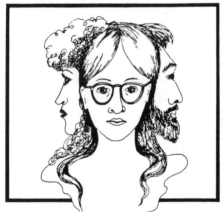

Multiple personality disorder stems from severe trauma early in life such as severe beatings or sexual abuse. The alternate personalities develop in response to the trauma to save the sanity of the individual. There may be many such alternate personalities of varying ages and of both sexes, in the same individual. The recognition of this mental disorder is relatively recent although the first case was reported in the German literature by Gmelin in 1791. He called it *exchange personality*. Hypnotherapy for these patients has become the prime method of treatment. The purpose is to integrate the various personalities into one whole being. Each personality can be contacted when the person is in a hypnotic trance. Therapy must be done by a psychiatrist well-trained in hypnotherapy. As a family physician, I have not been trained in this area of care and I would refer the patient to a psychotherapist with such training.

To understand a person with multiple personality disorder, let's consider our own minds. We are aware of our different personalities, referred to as *ego states* or subdivisions of the mind that are normal and natural. For example, at times I am performing in my role as family physician. The aura that goes with this ego state includes my professional manner, my concern for my patients and their families, and my relationships with my colleagues. I enter this ego state when I leave my home in the morning to see hospitalized patients. It continues through the day at my office and at times during the evening and night, if I am needed for further medical care.

When I am not working, however, and am at my cottage on the lake, I am a different person and am in a different ego state. I am playful, water-skiing with my kids and cooking out on the grill. My professional life is far from my mind. I am aware of my professional personality, however, and can revert to that mode if need be. I remember one occasion when a guest at the cottage fell and broke his arm. He asked if I could be his doctor for the injury although he was from another city and not my regular patient. I consented and immediately entered my professional ego state. When his arm had been set and the cast had been applied, we went back to the cottage and I again entered the role of relaxed host and he the role of a guest having as good a time as possible with a broken arm.

A third ego state that I sometimes enter is that of a

church musician. As a choir member and occasional church organist, I become quite saintly during church services. My religion should always be a part of my personality and I think that basically it is, but while in church, I feel and act different than while in other ego states.

In one ego state I may act in a particular circumstance as my father would have acted. In another, I might act as my mother might have acted. In yet another I might act like a friend or teacher. My foolhardy or fun-loving ego state comes from my childhood. All of these ego states are parts of my overall personality. I am aware of them and enter and leave them smoothly, but my conscious mind is always able to switch from one state to another.

The major difference between normal ego states and the various personalities of the patient with multiple personality disorder is that in the former the overall personality is aware of the various ego states. In the latter, each personality is independent and unaware of the others. The actions of people with multiple personality disorders cannot be predicted since their behavior depends on the personality in control at the time. People with normal personality integration will vary depending on the situation and which ego state he or she may be experiencing.

Hypnotherapy has become the prime form of therapy for multiple personality disorder. One patient's personalities may be entirely different from each other, with different voices and mannerisms, and sets of morals. For example, Suzie may be a successful businesswoman while Ann may be an immoral alcoholic, and Tom may be a macho TV sports addict while Gene may be a child who likes to play with dolls. All of these personalities may reside within one individual. There is usually a central *supreme personality* within the minds of these patients that is aware of all of the personalities. This central awareness can help the therapist in integrating the various personalities. Since different ages and sexes are involved, integration may take many years. During that time, the patient may have many psychological problems as each of the various personalities become aware of their condition. Some psychiatrists have devoted their professional careers to caring for these patients. Research is being conducted but much more must be known before therapy can be entirely satisfactory for these individuals. Interested readers are urged to explore the books on the subject such as *The Three Faces of Eve* and *Sybil*.

CHAPTER 14

Hypnosis for the Cancer Patient

Cancer is one of the most frightening words in our language. We all dread the possibility of developing cancer and shudder when we think about its consequences. Cancer is with us, however, and will continue to be a major cause of distress. In this chapter I will explore how hypnosis can benefit the cancer patient.

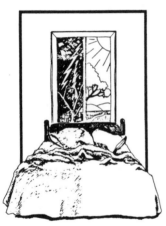

Keep in mind that cancer is not one individual disease. There are many forms and types of cancer. Many types can be cured by surgery. This is particularly true with certain types of skin cancer and cancers that are confined to a small area of an organ. Unfortunately, cancers tend to spread, and a surgeon is not able to remove all cancer cells when they spread to other areas of the body. Certain medicines kill cancer cells, and some cancers such as leukemia respond well to this chemotherapy. Unfortunately, chemotherapy has undesirable side effects. While killing the cancer cells, the medicines also injure normal cells. This causes patient discomfort. Radiation therapy is being used more and more to treat cancer patients. Again, there are side effects. Cancer research is continuing at a rapid rate, and new forms of therapy are constantly being discovered. Combinations of surgery, chemotherapy and radiation therapy are frequently used.

Hypnotherapy is a useful form of treatment for the cancer patient. First, it gives the patient a feeling of control. The patient needs to be treated by specialists trained in the treatmentl of cancer, but frequently the specialist tells the patient what must be done and leaves the patient feeling out of control. This feeling is heightened if the cancer patient requires hospitalization. With self-hypnosis he or she can regain a feeling of control over the situation. Hypnosis can aid in the lessening of discomfort of the cancer directly by pain-relieving suggestions. It can lessen the nausea and vomiting associated with chemotherapy. It can help the patient relax during radiation therapy. Feelings of helplessness and hopelessness can be diminished.

While these types of suggestions are aimed at comfort, there is also evidence that the patient may be able to attack the cancer directly through thought processes. The 25th Commemorative Volume of the American Journal of Clinical Hypnosis is devoted entirely to hypnosis and cancer.* Several articles in that volume give striking evidence that the subconscious mind does influence the immune system, which can attack cancer cells directly. Most physicians now believe that we all produce cancer cells from time to time and that our immune systems destroy them before they have a chance to develop into full-blown cancer. This theory can explain why some people have spontaneous cures of proven cancer. It may also explain some of the "miraculous" cures we read about.

Hypnotherapy uses the subconscious part of the mind to control sensation and movement. Preliminary studies indicate that the subconscious can also influence the immune system. It seems reasonable that

---

* *American Journal of Clinical Hypnosis,* Volume 25 , Numbers 2-3, October 1982-January 1983.

hypnotherapy may be help a person control the growth and spread of cancer.

Everyone with cancer who is capable of concentrating on an idea can be helped with hypnosis. We must foster its use to an ever greater extent. Everyone who needs this type of therapy should have access to it. A case study taken from my own files will serve as an example of use of hypnotherapy for a patient with cancer.

J.S. had both breasts removed for cancer seven years before I saw her. Her cancer had spread to her liver. Her cancer doctor asked me to see her while she was undergoing further therapy. She was scheduled to be hospitalized for the insertion of a tube into the arteries of the liver so that cancer medicines could be introduced directly into the substance of the liver. She was a single 54-year-old woman who had had a phobia since childhood about nausea and vomiting. She was afraid of anything that might cause nausea. For example, she would not ride in a boat for fear of seasickness. She was warned that the liver treatment was likely to cause nausea, so she refused the treatment. I saw J.S. in my office to explore the use of hypnosis. She was well read regarding suggestion therapy and seemed eager to pursue it. She was an average hypnotic subject but was highly motivated. I taught her self-hypnosis and instructed her to practice several times each day. I gave her suggestions that would help her learn to accept any mild stomach upset that might accompany her therapy. I stressed the need for the health-giving medicines that would help fight the cancer cells and urged her to develop a positive attitude toward her therapy. I next visited J.S. while she was a patient in the hospital. I saw her on two occasions a week apart. I reinforced the suggestions that I had given her before. She had 11 days of chemotherapy directly into the liver with a minimum of discomfort and no vomiting. She was very enthusiastic about the relative ease of the therapy although she had developed some dryness of the lips and a few sores in her mouth. Her cancer specialist chose to discontinue therapy for a few days because of the mouth sores. He stated that her lack of nausea and vomiting were rare since most patients with mouth sores complained of nausea and vomiting. Although J.S. eventually died of her disease, she was able to live her last weeks free of discomfort despite her intensive chemotherapy.

Another example of the use of hypnotherapy in a cancer patient was discussed in Chapter 8. In that case the problem was severe pain which responded to suggestions of the pleasant surroundings of her flower garden. Other examples would include the use of hypnotherapy for allaying the depression accompanying the knowledge of having cancer and continuing to enjoy life to the fullest extent possible.

CHAPTER 15

Dangers and Limitations
of Medical Hypnosis

Hypnosis is safe. It is safer than penicillin or aspi-
rin. There are, however, some cautions. It is a very
powerful tool and must be used by a trained therapist.

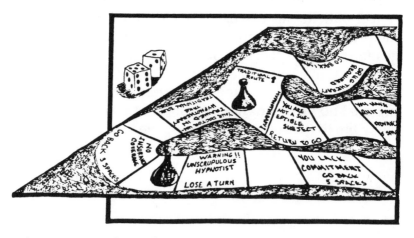

Anyone can be a hypnotist since it is easy to learn
what to say. The hypnotist is essentially a teacher and
the hypnotic subject is the one who actually hypnotizes himself or herself. An unscrupulous person may
hypnotize a willing and susceptible subject and offer
suggestions related to performing acts which would
be immoral or illegal. The subject has the power to resist, but if he or she has no moral reason to resist, the
suggestions may be acted upon. Some hypnotists believe that it is possible for a person to hypnotize another person and actually cause him to commit
crimes. Studies are being conducted to help determine

whether this is possible.

A patient with a severe mental problem may have an adverse reaction to hypnosis. I stopped therapy for a migraine patient when she became very agitated upon entering a trance, stating that she felt she was falling into a deep hole. There were obviously deep psychological implications which I felt unprepared to handle. I continued to care for her in the more traditional medical manner.

If hypnosis is so great, why aren't all doctors using it? This is a question which I am frequently asked. For most patients, hypnosis is still on the fringe of acceptance. It conjures up hocus pocus and voodoo. It brings to mind the stage hypnotist who uses it for entertainment. It seems too good to be true. In many instances, it is too good to be true. It simply doesn't always work. Scientific reports regarding hypnosis for quitting smoking range from practically no success to 97% success. A few years ago I studied 83 of my smoking patients and found that 25% of them were nonsmokers after a year following a single, one hour hypnosis visit. These results are somewhat discouraging, but for the 21 patients who became permanent nonsmokers it may well have been the difference between life and death. Hypnosis is not like surgery where something that is diseased is cut out. It requires the motivation and cooperation of the patient. It is simply a means by which a patient can use his or her subconscious in a constructive way for a specific problem. The hypnotherapist is a teacher who trains the patient in the technique, but the patient needs to use it for his or her own benefit.

Hypnosis for chronic pain is useful only in the context of a team approach. Physical therapy, nutrition, family therapy and mechanical devices are also needed. Chemical anesthesia is so successful, hypnosis really isn't needed except in the rare occasion when a patient is allergic to the usual chemical anesthetic agents. Hypnosis allows the patient to assume control over functions, feelings, attitudes and activities which a person had no previous control. It gives time outs from suffering, changes in habits and new attitudes toward life.

Hypnotic techniques are not taught in our medical schools. If they are mentioned at all, they are usually referred to in a psychiatry lecture or seminar. A few medical schools do foster its use. They tend to be schools at which certain faculty members have become interested in the topic and are doing research on hypnosis. Usually the individual practitioner must find the time and effort to learn medical hypnosis on his or her own.

My experiences with hypnosis began when several of my patients asked me to learn about it. If it is to be used more extensively, it will be because patients request it.

Should we continue to foster its use? Should we continue to do research on it? Should we as patients demand that our doctors learn more about it? Yes, we should. There is plenty of evidence that medical hypnosis is of great value to a large number of patients. There probably won't be a time when every doctor is trained to use hypnosis, but its use will gradually increase as more patients demand it and more doctors become interested in learning about it.

CHAPTER 16

The Future of Medical Hypnosis

Hypnosis in Sports

Hypnosis has a place in sports and physical fitness. Athletes have been "psyched up" for greater performance over the centuries by "pep talks" but seldom have there been well planned methods for increasing physical performance.

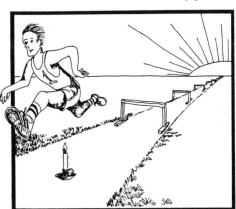

The extent to which hypnosis is used in sports is difficult to evaluate. Questionnaires have been sent to athletic directors but the returns have been scanty and not dependable. There are reports of the routine use of autogenic techniques (which are similar to hypnosis) by sport psychologists in Czechoslovakia and Australia. These techniques are used for precompetition anxiety. Similar applications of hypnosis have been reported in work with American, British, and Japanese athletes.

People are capable of greater physical exertion than they ordinarily exhibit. The super strength needed to lift a car which has pinned a child or the broken bones which can accompany electric shock therapy testify to strength that is available and not often used. We are partially limited in what we do by pain, which is a protective mechanism. We may not be able to unscrew a glass jar, not because we don't have the strength, but because it hurts beyond a certain level of acceptance. The athlete learns to endure the pain and achieve despite it, but there is a point where actual damage to tissue occurs.

Physicians, coaches and trainers must use caution when attempting greater physical performance from athletes by psychological means, however, because there are certain dangers. First, there is a danger of causing physical damage to the body. Stress fractures, shin splints, hemorrhage within muscles and dislocated joints are examples of the consequences of excessive activity. The reduction of pain through hypnosis can remove the naturally protective device that protects our bodies. Second, over-emphasis on the importance of winning may cause poor eating habits. An example is the high school boy who wishes to stay in a particular weight class for wrestling and actually harms his body by his eating habits. Hypnosis has nothing to do with over-stressing the importance of sports and it should not be used in an attempt to exceed the limits of the body of the participant. Hypnosis is useful, however, in helping athletes relax and in removing anxieties which may be detrimental to their performance.

Studies indicate that negative suggestions designed to decrease muscular performance are far more likely to be effective than positive suggestions designed to increase performance. There are reports that hypnosis prior to a performance does indeed improve an athlete's performance. Other studies, however, show that there are no effects. Surely there is room for more study of these effects. Relaxation can be enhanced. Motivation can be enhanced. Whether actual physical performance can be enhanced is still open to question. Hypnosis and other forms of "mind altering" are very complex. As yet, there is no proof that these forms of psychotherapy consistently affect athletic performance. For the casual exerciser or fitness bug, however, hypnosis can be useful for keeping him or her motivated to exercise. Further research along these lines may uncover uses and effects as yet unknown.

Hypnosis in General Education

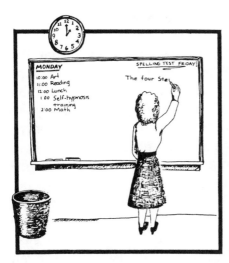

Some workers in the field of hypnosis feel that everyone should have the knowledge and ability to use self-hypnosis. Should self-hypnosis be taught as routine skill in grade school, much like learning to add and read? Since hypnosis is easy to learn and is useful for relaxation in times of stress, and since people vary in their ability to enter the trance state, should we not be determining susceptibility and training everyone in self-hypnosis? I feel that we should. We should include relaxation techniques at an early level in schooling. Studies have shown that children between the ages of seven and eleven are the most susceptible, but five year olds can also benefit from training in hypnosis.

One potential drawback to teaching hypnosis in the

schools is that teachers may gain too much influence over the children. A poor teacher, or an unscrupulous one, might influence students negatively if allowed to use hypnotic techniques. Specially trained teachers, therefore, should do the teaching.

An experiment in Japan revealed another negative aspect of this approach. Teenage girls were taught hypnotic techniques and used them as they might use drugs, to get a psychological "high." This would be safer than actually using drugs, but the consequences might be to the student's disadvantage.

Hypnosis and the Immune System

Medical teachers tend to foster the idea that the mind and the body are not directly related. The surgeon may be excellent with the knife, but he may cause the patient mental hardship by what he says to the patient, either before or after surgery. Whether his words actually influence the healing process is speculative at this time. Norman Cousins has written several excellent books about the healing relationship between the mind and the body. Studies indicate that the mind influences the immune system. The immune system controls the bodies ability to fight off disease whether it be in the form of viruses, bacteria or even cancer cells. The concept of 'psychosurgery' is the idea that positive thoughts can remove diseased tissue. I assume this to mean that the mind can increase natural resistance to disease. Although it is in its early stages of development, there is enough evidence of its value to foster further study. The future of immunology may well parallel the future of medical hypnosis.

I like to envision a future where all physicians, teachers, and parents have the ability to use hypnosis for their patients, students and children. Although suggestion therapy has been around for centuries, the many opportunities for psychotherapy using hypnotic techniques are only beginning to be realized.

Society must always be alert to the misuse of such potent forces, however, because mass hypnosis can be devastating. Adolph Hitler, a master hypnotist, is an example of a man who had an understanding of mind control which he used with disastrous results. The potential uses of hypnosis, yoga, transcendental meditation, relaxation techniques, La Maze and other uses of the trance state require further study and development. Perhaps in the next several decades, we can overcome our prejudices against these techniques. Perhaps we can encourage—and demand—their greater use.

CHAPTER 17

Medical Hypnosis: A Summary

This book is but a brief introduction to medical hypnosis. I have discussed some of its uses in general medicine and in the realm of psychology. Although suggestion therapy has been around for centuries, only within the last 200 years has it come under the scrutiny of scientific investigation. The scientific inves-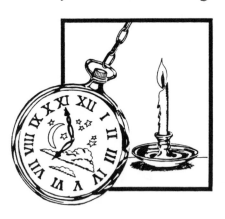tigation of the mind has always had hazards since there are nearly infinite variables which must be considered.

Most reports in the medical literature regarding hypnosis are anecdotes which tell of varying degrees of success using varying types of suggestion. When subjected to controlled scientific investigation, hypnosis stands up as a useful but highly confusing form of treatment. There are many scientific studies underway regarding medical hypnosis. Many fine investigators are tackling the problems related to the study of the mind.

What can hypnosis do for you? If you have insomnia, if you are a smoker, if you have a phobia such as fear of flying, if you have a chronic pain problem, if you are going to have a baby and if you fit into countless other categories, you can benefit from medical hypnosis.

Where do you go to get this form of therapy? At this time there are very limited numbers of physicians, psychologists, psychiatrists and dentists who use hypnosis on a routine basis. Even though it is accepted as a reasonable form of therapy by the major medical and dental organizations throughout the world, it has not become part of mainstream medical practice. You should check with local medical or dental organizations to find doctors and dentists who use hypnosis. You can also contact the American Society of Clinical Hypnosis for a listing of doctors who have taken courses through its educational branch. You can read more books on the subject. There are many books available written at varying levels of complexity. I have listed some examples of further reading at the back of this book.

Let's hope that medical hypnosis will become more and more available as scientific enquiry continues to advance.

Suggested Reading

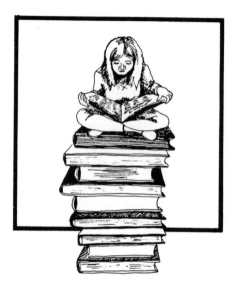

Barber, Theodore X., Spanos, Nicholas P., Chaves, John F.: *Hypnotism, Imagination, and Human Potentialities*. Pergamon Press. 1974.

The traditional explanation of hypnotism is criticized in this book. Five basic assumptions of hypnosis, many of which are described in this book, are considered to be inaccurate by these authors. It is written for the professional and is heavy reading for the non-scientist, but the concepts are interesting. There are two appendices which discuss The Barber Suggestibility Scale and Surgery with Acupuncture which are of note.

Bernstein, Morey, *The Search for Bridey Murphy*. Doubleday & Company, Inc. 1965.

Although this is not a book primarily about hypnosis,

it is interesting in that hypnosis is extensively used. Mr. Bernstein describes his use of hypnosis with Ruth Simmons on several occasions. He takes her back in time to a previous life, that of an Irish woman, Bridey Murphy McCarthy. The book contains excellent Appendices regarding hypnosis in general and more specifically hypnosis in medicine, hypnotizability, age regression, post hypnotic suggestion, extrasensory perception, clairvoyance, psychokinesis and parapsychology.

Block, Eugene B., *Hypnosis: A New Tool in Crime Detection.* **David McKay Co., 1976.**

This book discusses the history of hypnosis as it relates to crime detection. It describes a number of interesting criminal cases where hypnosis was used.

Bowers, Kenneth S. *Hypnosis for the Seriously Curious.* **W. W. Norton & Company, 1976.**

This book's prime purpose is to seek the answers to the puzzling and elusive phenomenon known as hypnosis. It is written for the professional, but is quite understandable to the non-scientist. It contains a large bibliography.

Caprio, Frank S. M.D., Berger, Joseph R. *Helping Yourself With Self-Hypnosis.* **Warner Books. 1963.**

This book was written for the non-scientist and, although dated, still offers a good comprehensive overview of hypnosis. It contains many self-help ideas which can enhance a persons life.

Dauven, Jean, *The Powers of Hypnosis*. A Scarborough Book, Stein and Day. 1965. (Translated from the French by Joyce E. Clemow).

This book is rather unique in that it gives a French view of the history of hypnosis and its application. The author discusses the history of hypnosis in some detail with a fascinating account of Dr. Mesmer and his twenty seven propositions. It also gives brief biographies of the important persons working with hypnosis prior to the 1960s. This book is easy and entertaining reading for the non-scientist.

Erickson, Milton H., M.D., Hershman, Seymour, M.D., Secter, Irving I., D.D.S., *The Practical Application of Medical and Dental Hypnosis*. The Julian Press, Inc. 1961.

This classic book on hypnosis includes many case studies of Dr. Erickson and is fascinating reading for those interested in case studies. It accurately reveals Ericksonian hypnotic techniques.

Gill, Merton M. M.D., Brenman, Margaret, Ph.D.: *Hypnosis and Related States, Psychoanalytic Studies in Regression*. International Universities Press, Inc. New York. 1959.

Rather outdated, but a good review of hypnosis in general for the time it was written. It includes induction, the hypnotic state, theory of induction and the hypnotic state, the metapsychology of regression and hypnosis, somnambulism, fugue states, brain-washing, trance in Bali and explorations of the use of hypnosis in psychotherapy. It has a large bibliography.

Haley, Jay, *Uncommon Therapy*. Ballantine Books, New York 1973.

This book provides an excellent account of Dr. Milton H. Erickson, one of the founders of modern medical hypnosis. Mr. Haley describes in great detail the methods of Dr. Erickson and uses many case studies to illustrate his information.

Hilgard, Ernest R., *Hypnotic Susceptibility*. Harcourt Brace Jovanovich, Inc. 1965.

This book is the standard text relative to hypnotic susceptibility. It contains a scientific explanation of methods to determine susceptibility and is not for the casual reader. Since it is one of the classics in the field, however, I felt I should include it in this list.

Hilgard, Ernest R., Hilgard, Josephine R. *Hypnosis in the Relief of Pain*. William Kaufmann, Inc. 1975.

This classic in hypnosis literature presents scientific proof of the value of medical hypnosis in pain relief. It also discusses the clinical use of hypnosis for patients with acute and chronic pain.

Hilgard, Josephine R., M.D. *Personality and Hypnosis, A Study of Imaginative Involvement*, Second Edition. The University of Chicago Press, Chicago and London. 1979.

This book details scientific evidence supporting the concept that observation of certain personality traits can predict hypnotizibility. It was written for the professional, but the hardy reader would find the concepts to be very interesting.

LeCron, Leslie M., *Self Hypnotism: The Technique and Its Use in Daily Living*. Prentice-Hall, Inc. 1964.

This is a "How To Do It Book" regarding self hypnosis. It includes various self-tests to help you learn more about your own personality and what you can do to make some changes.

LeCron, Leslie M., *The Complete Guide to Hypnosis*. Harper & Row, Publishers 1971.

Here is a book which gives an easy to read comprehensive account of medical hypnosis. It includes a chapter on self-hypnosis which gives a lucid account of the use of hypnosis by the individual.

Pratt, George J., PhD., Wood, Dennis P. Ph.D., Alman, Brian M., Ph.D. *A Clinical Hypnosis Primer*. Psychology & Consulting Associates Press. 1984.

This book is written for professionals but it is within the grasp of the well educated non-scientific person. I found it to be a fascinating book and one that is well worth reading.

Shor, Ronald E. Orne, Martin T., *The Nature of Hypnosis: Selected Basic Readings*. Holt, Rinehart and Winston, Inc. 1965.

Although this book was compiled in 1965, it contains 34 selected writings by the leaders in hypnosis. There are original articles by Franz Anton Mesmer, Ronald Shor, Milton H. Erickson, Pierre Janet, and well as many others. For basic knowledge of the field, this book stands out as a winner.

Straus, Roger A., Ph.D., *Strategic Self Hypnosis.* **Prentice-Hall, Inc. 1982.**

This book is an excellent "do it yourself" handbook on the use of self-hypnosis. It explains clearly in non-professional terms how to use self-hypnosis to overcome stress, improve performance and live to ones fullest potential.

Wain, Harold J., Ph.D., *Clinical Hypnosis in Medicine.* **Symposia Specialists, Inc. 1980.**
Dr. Wain has written a chapter in this book on the use of hypnosis in chronic pain. He also edited the remaining chapters covering many aspects of medical hypnosis. It is a scientific book but the non-scientist might find it to be of interest.

Wilson, Ian, *All In The Mind.* **Doubleday & Company, Inc. 1982.**

A further investigation of reincarnation with a detailed analysis of many purported cases makes up the content of this book. Mr. Wilson explains many cases of "reincarnation" as a type of multiple personality. He does not, however completely debunk the concept. It is an interesting book and written for the average reader.

Wolberg, Lewis R. M.D. *Hypnosis: Is It for You?* **Harcourt Brace Jovanovich, Inc. 1972.**

Dr. Wolberg has written a highly readable scientific book about hypnosis. It is for the inquisitive person who wishes to expand his or her knowledge about this subject.

Wyckoff, James, Franz Anton Mesmer, *Between God and Devil*. Prentice-Hall, Inc. 1975.

Quite a number of books have been written about Franz Anton Mesmer. This highly readable book outlines this remarkable man's life and interests. The reader will find it to be a good foundation for Mesmer's contribution to the study of hypnosis prior to the 1960s. This book is easy and entertaining reading.

Appendix

For further information regarding medical hypnosis
you may contact the following organizations:

American Society of Clinical Hypnosis
2250 E. Devon Avenue
Suite 336
Des Plaines, IL   60018
(708) 297-3317

Society of Clinical and Experimental Hypnosis
128-A Kings Park Drive
Liverpool, NY   13090
(315) 652-7299

Milton H. Erickson Foundation
3606 N. 24th Street
Phoenix, AZ   85016-6500
(602) 956-6196

International Society of Hypnosis
Department of Psychiatry
University of Melbourne
Austin Hospital
Heidelberg, Victoria
Australia   3084
(613) 459-6499

Index